Umida Babazhanova

Affective-respiratory paroxysm in children and issues of treatment tactics

Umida Babazhanova

Affective-respiratory paroxysm in children and issues of treatment tactics

Monograph

ScienciaScripts

Imprint

Cover image: www.ingimage.com

This book is a translation from the original published under ISBN 978-620-8-17245-9.

Publisher:
Sciencia Scripts
is a trademark of
Dodo Books Indian Ocean Ltd. and OmniScriptum S.R.L publishing group

120 High Road, East Finchley, London, N2 9ED, United Kingdom
Str. Armeneasca 28/1, office 1, Chisinau MD-2012, Republic of Moldova, Europe
Printed at: see last page
ISBN: 978-620-8-28867-9

MINISTRY OF HEALTH OF THE REPUBLIC OF UZBEKISTAN

On the rights of the manuscript

УДК:616.853-009.24-053:616.07

UMIDA TAZHIMURATOVNA BABAZHANOVA

AFFECTIVE-RESPIRATORY PAROXYSM IN CHILDREN AND ISSUES OF TREATMENT TACTICS

14.00.13-Neurology

MONOGRAPHY.

Tashkent-2024

CONTENTS.

INTRODUCTION

Affective-respiratory paroxysm (ARP) is one of the frequently observed non-epileptic paroxysmal disorders (NEPDs) in young children, manifested by involuntary breath-holding with brief impairment of consciousness and motor activity in response to exogenous stimuli. These qualities are also described in actual epileptic seizures. According to the World Health Organisation, "...epilepsy is misdiagnosed in 40 per cent of the total population"[1] . The relevance of ARP is determined by the high risk of its transformation into epileptic seizures, as well as its negative impact on neuropsychiatric development. Identification of clinical features, etiology, pathogenesis and risk factors in patients with NEPS, prevention of unjustified prescription of long-term antiepileptic therapy and improvement of patients' quality of life is one of the urgent problems in the medical field.

In the world, research is being conducted to identify childhood problems, their early diagnosis and achieving a highly effective approach to treatment tactics. In this regard, the identification of causes, risk factors of affective-respiratory paroxysms in children, factors of development and prevention of complications of the disease, elimination of neuropsychological, neurovegetative maladaptation, identification of biochemical disorders at the onset of the disease, as well as the improvement of treatment and prevention methods are recognised as an urgent problem. The clinical and neurological approach to the development of a set of measures aimed at optimising early diagnosis, treatment and prevention of

[1] OWH.World report on ageingand health:World Health Organisation 2016

complications taking into account biochemical changes in children with ARP acquires a special meaning.

In our country, extensive measures are being taken to develop the medical sphere according to world standards, in particular for early diagnosis and to reduce complications of neurological diseases among various segments of the population. Important tasks aimed at "...prevention and diagnosis of diseases, introduction of high-tech methods, provision of highly qualified and quality medical care" have been defined[2] . These tasks are one of the most urgent scientific directions for early detection of non-epileptic paroxysmal conditions in children and implementation of measures aimed at preventing complications, increasing the completeness of medical and social care for children and reducing disability rates, as well as improving the quality of life.

The work of many scientists is devoted to optimising the diagnosis of affective-respiratory paroxysms using high-tech research methods (Stephenson J.B.P., 2003; Khura D.S., Valencia I., Kruthiventi S., et al., 2006; Francis J. DiMario Jr, 2009). The cause of the development of ARP is unknown, but it has been found to be inherited in an autosomal type with reduced penetrance. (Walsh M et al., 2012). Several studies have implicated autonomic dysfunction, delayed myelination in the medulla oblongata and iron deficiency anaemia in the pathogenesis of ARP (Olsen A.L., 2010; Kelly A.M., 2014; Porter C.J., 2016; Espinosa R.E., 2017). Serum selenium and superoxide dismutase levels have been found to be reduced in patients with ARP, which is an important pathogenetic factor in

---

[2]Decree of the President of the Republic of Uzbekistan No. UP 5590 "On comprehensive measures to radically improve the health care system of the Republic of Uzbekistan" dated 7 December 2018.

disease progression (Khaled Saad et al., 2014). The imbalance of the antioxidant system and the role of lipid peroxidation (LPO) in the development of epileptic conditions have been identified (Kodirova A.Sh., 2011). Implantable pacemakers have been used to treat severe, prolonged episodes of ARP associated with life-threatening bradycardia or asystole (Kelly 2001).

Studies have reported that patients with febrile and afebrile seizures had decreased melatonin levels after seizures (Dabak et al., 2019). The antioxidant and neurometabolic properties of melatonin were also found to have positive effects on children with epilepsy (Ross et al., 2018). The anticonvulsant effects of melatonin have been found to inhibit GAMK a receptors in pyramidal cells (Stewart wa Liyun, 2021). In the treatment of epilepsy, the addition of melatonin to the complex treatment of patients aged 8 months to 18 years has been shown to reduce epileptic seizures (Hancock et al., 2005). Melatonin can serve as a potential therapeutic scavenger of free radicals (hydroxyl radicals, hydrogen peroxide, singlet oxygen) and a broad-spectrum antioxidant (activation of antioxidant pathways; superoxide dismutase, catalase, glutathione peroxidase, glutathione reductase) (Wade A. G., 2010).

Currently, scientific studies are being conducted to determine the degree of correlation between biochemical changes in pathology, despite the high incidence of affective-respiratory paroxysms in early childhood. In particular, in the development of affective-respiratory paroxysms in children, it is important to identify risk factors, determine pathogenetic, clinical-neurophysiological and neuroimaging features, develop diagnostic criteria, eliminate ARP attacks, correct biochemical disorders and prevent complications caused by this pathology, use modern diagnostic capabilities, improve the effectiveness of treatment and preventive measures.

CHAPTER I. AFFECTIVE-RESPIRATORY PAROXYSMS: A REVIEW OF THE LITERATURE

§1.1 Clinical problem and epidemiology of affective-respiratory paroxysms

Non-epileptic paroxysmal states (NEPs) are clinical disorders, usually sudden-onset, short-lived cerebral dysfunction from a variety of causes with a general non-epileptic character. Non-epileptic paroxysmal conditions are more common than epileptic conditions. NEPS can be confused with epileptic seizures. These conditions manifest themselves through tremors, stereotyped movements in wakefulness or difficult to explain states in sleep. These phenomena are difficult to diagnose unequivocally as normal, pathological, or adaptive. These states are currently defined as paroxysms (***Paroxysm,*** (spets. and scrib.). *A sudden and violent attack (of a disease, feeling). (Explanatory Dictionary ed. by S.I. Ozhegov and N.Y. Shvedova).*

Current epidemiological studies show that in the first year of life, epilepsy occurs in 50-200 cases out of 100,000 children, with non-epileptic events in this cohort reaching 60-70% [53: 919-921-c].

Non-epileptic paroxysms are very difficult to distinguish from epileptic seizures. This is because the clinical and neurological signs of NEPS are also seen in epileptic seizures. It is impossible to differentiate an epileptic phenomenon from a non-epileptic phenomenon on first assessment. It is also possible for individual children to have more than one phenomenon. The correct approach to diagnosis is a thorough history and examination, and this will result in most cases in an accurate resolution of the problem. Periodic observation will give the clinician ample opportunity to gather extensive clinical data on the subject in question. Because of differences in age and maturity level or the presence of additional underlying neurological abnormalities, additional information or descriptive embellishments are often lacking. In some respects, this allows for a clearer observation of what is going on. However, in these circumstances, much of what we are trying to answer in our conversation with the patient and individualised description of symptoms may go unanswered or misinterpreted. Recognition of misdiagnosis, especially of epilepsy, in these populations (infants, young children and children with neurological impairment) can be significant [92: 234-240-c]. An even more important concept is that there may be ambiguity and clinical uncertainty for any particular diagnosis of epilepsy or non-epileptic seizure [30: 155-161-c]. Misdiagnosis of epilepsy is recognised worldwide and may be more problematic when made by non-specialists. In some population-based studies, the ratio of misdiagnosis to correct diagnosis has been found to be as high as 3: 1.28. The "uncertain" diagnostic category has been reported to range from 0% to 24% [46:704-706-c].

There have been at least seven large studies identifying these problems [65:477-480-c]. Initial diagnosis of epilepsy, after referral, 16-33% of study subjects were found to have specific non-epileptic paroxysmal disorders [51:585-589-c].

Several population-based studies have provided a better understanding of the frequency of misdiagnosis of epilepsy and data on the prevalence of non-epileptic paroxysmal events [65:477-480-

c]. The overall condition of the patient is a core category of clinical medicine. The founder of Developmental Neurology, H.F. R. Precht (2017), believes that determining the status of the nervous system as required by the sequence of neurological examinations is an important component of the examination. This is especially true in developing children, and assessing their condition in these children is challenging due to the presence of poorly differentiated and difficult to interpret phenomena in children of this age [14:136-c].

A frequently observed non-epileptic paroxysmal condition in young children is affective-respiratory paroxysms (ARP), manifested by involuntary apnoea with short-term impairment of consciousness and motor activity in response to a provoking factor. In modern practice, ARP leads to misdiagnosis of epilepsy due to similar paroxysmal conditions (loss of consciousness, apnoea, cyanosis, sometimes the presence of tonic and convulsive spasms). It should be noted that ARPs do not occur only in healthy children; they can occur in organic lesions of the CNS or in epilepsy, which presents certain difficulties in differential diagnosis [44:265-269-c].

Such paroxysmal cases in young children were known centuries ago since the time of Hippocrates ("In an attack of breath-holding, the child suddenly stops breathing as a result of mysterious terror or fear of other people's cries, or during crying, in which the blood supply to the brain is reduced, the child becomes pale and loses consciousness.") [88: 354-361-c], but the first description in scientific literature was written by Nicholas Culpepper (1616-1654): ("Children have this disease .... On account of anger or sorrow the heart moves from the centre to the diaphragm and breathing stops, when the provoking factor ceases, these symptoms also disappear.")") [22:561-565-c]. Furthermore, in the nineteenth and early twentieth century, their clinical features were described in detail, which were later labelled infantile form of hysteria or infantile syncope by Rill and Barthesin in 1843 and by Meigsin in 1848.

In the 20th century, various authors published their clinical views on their pathophysiological and prognostic significance. To this end, various terms and definitions have been used to refer to the relevant paroxysmal episodes in infants and young children.

The term "breath-holding attacks" or "reflex anoxic attacks" is currently used in much of the English-language literature. However, D. D. Korostovtsev et al. authors (2007) introduced the term "affective-respiratory seizures" into Russian neuropediatrics, as this definition describes the involuntary presence of a preceding stimulus (fear, pain, dread), as well as the sequential and involuntary development of symptoms (respiratory disturbance, apnoea, seizure, disharmony) [14:59-61-c].

ARP occurs mainly in children under 5-6 years of age. The debut most often occurs between 6 and 18 months of age (up to 80%). In about 15% of cases, first seizure-like episodes occur in infants under 6 months of age, rarely even in the first weeks or months, and in children in less than 2% of cases after 10 years of age. ARP is identified at least once in 5-6% of children aged 3-17 years [14:62-c]. It should be noted that the actual prevalence of ARP may be even more important, as in some cases parents who are aware of this paroxysmal condition in children do not consult specialists for this problem because of single, infrequent attacks. The frequency of ARP in a child varies widely, from several times a day (once a day), to a single episode or several episodes per year. However, it is indicated that the average frequency of seizures at onset and during the active period is 1-5 per week. Generally, after the onset of an attack, their frequency increases and then decreases. According to epidemiological studies, ARP, like many other neurological diseases, occurs in boys at about a ratio of 1.3 to 1.5 than in girls [40:547-550-c]. However, in the daily practice of the paediatric neurologist, it sometimes seems that the opposite proportions - the predominance of ARP - are observed in girls [21]. The family history of such paroxysms is aggravated in 23-38% of cases and at the same time in epilepsy does not exceed population averages [58: 129-130-c]. Maternal family dominance suggests a possible additional role of genomic imprinting. The reported prevalence of severe ARP ranges from 0.1 to 4.6%. However, a focused survey of relatives shows higher rates of ARP approaching the maximum (14.6%) [102: 295-300-c].

Pathogenetic mechanisms of development and clinical manifestations of paroxysms allow us to distinguish, first of all, on the basis of changes in the skin of the child's face during an attack - "cyanotic" (CARP) and "pale" (BARP), as well as "mixed" (ARP). The distribution of ARP by skin changes is BARP 61% -78%, CARP 25% - 36%, and ATS 26-46%. Taking into account the main clinical and pathogenetic differences between the seizures Stevenson (1978) distinguished these fundamentally different nosological types and proposed the use of the term - "reflex anoxic seizure" [14:59-61-c].

§1.2 Etiopathogenesis of affective-respiratory paroxysms in young children.

Affective-respiratory paroxysm (ARP), as the name suggests, is an episode in which a child involuntarily stops breathing and briefly loses consciousness immediately after a frightening or emotionally upsetting event or after a painful experience. The diagnosis is based primarily on the nature of the initial provocation that causes the child emotional discomfort (apnoea, colour change (pale or cyanotic) and loss of consciousness). According to its clinical course, ARP is divided into mild, moderate and severe forms. Mild ARP is completed after colour change and difficulty in breathing. The severe form of ARP is accompanied by progressive postural tonus and impaired consciousness. The child often assumes an opisthotonus position and short myoclonic contractions may be observed. When the seizures stop, there is a period of relief and sighing.

ARP develops not only in healthy born children, but also as a result of perinatal damage to the central nervous system, which leads to difficulties in diagnosis and differential diagnosis.

There are several factors in the development of ARP: genetic predisposition, dysregulation of the autonomic nervous system and delayed myelination of the brainstem. Anaemia and iron deficiency have previously been associated with ARP, although the pathogenetic mechanism is still unclear. In addition, ARP can sometimes be the initial symptom of QT interval prolongation syndrome or paroxysmal cardiac rhythm disturbances. Therefore, electrocardiography (ECG) is recommended for QT interval prolongation syndrome. Associated myoclonic twitches after crying episodes may be seen with marked attacks of pallor and, to a lesser extent, with attacks of cyanotic behaviour. [17:61-65-c].

In the middle of the last century, researchers in their scientific work suggested that hereditary predisposition plays a role in the development of ARP. 20-30% of cases are inherited in the autosomal dominant type [101:1528-1167-c].

Autonomic dysregulation is a common physiological mechanism for the development of affective-respiratory paroxysms. It appears to be maturation-dependent, with gradual resolution of this propensity for dysregulation over time. Reflex sympathetic hyperactivity is associated with sinus attacks, and reflex parasympathetic hyperactivity is associated with pale attacks [36:351-359-c]. Early studies of autonomic responses were prompted by the observation of a parent who noted a slowing of her infant's heart rate during the pale period [83:5-22-c]. Many investigators have studied the oculocardial reflex using ocular compression. Simultaneous pressure on both closed eyeballs for 10 seconds triggers afferent signals via the ocular branch of the trigeminal nerve back to the cardiac motor bodies of the brainstem vagus nerves. This, in turn, leads to rapid efferent signalling via the vagus nerve to the sinoatrial node of the heart, resulting in cardiac slowing or transient asystole and prolongation of the R-R interval. The intention was to induce syncope or anoxic seizure for diagnostic purposes; however, asystole of more than 2 seconds was often used as a positive test. Stephenson reviewed the normative data and observed responses in detail. A period of asystole >6 seconds is required to achieve >98%

specificity and sensitivity. It can be questioned whether there is currently any clinical application to simply induce asystole during EEG recording [27:1150-c]. If the procedure does not induce an anoxic seizure that is recognisable as the exact type of event the parents observed, the procedure becomes largely an academic exercise. If the result is a confirmed event, the diagnostic validity of syncope can be assured. This centrally mediated parasympathetic stimulus is more readily elicited in children with vagal mediated ARP (i.e., pale type ARP), but can also be elicited in patients with cyanotic ARP. A more recent study in 116 patients with ARP compared to 46 patients with epilepsy were analysed retrospectively [92:234-240-c]. The authors used the duration of asystole for 2 seconds as a positive response and found that there was only 26% sensitivity in patients with epilepsy, but found 100% specificity in ARP [92:234-240-c]. Of course, both epilepsy and syncope can occur simultaneously in the same child. It is similar in that many children show mixed patterns of ARP, that is, either the cyanotic or pale type predominates, but both types are expressed at different times or in some unspecified combination of the two at the same time.

The basic pathophysiology of ARP involves interactions between CNS maturity, respiratory control mechanisms, cardiopulmonary mechanisms, blood oxygen capacity, and the autonomic nervous system. CARP as a type 1 hypoxic crisis and BARP as a type 2 hypoxic crisis, that each type can occur in the same child [93-:49-56-c]. The main conclusions to be drawn from these studies are that there is a strong propensity for reflex asystole via the vagal mechanism.

In the classic work by Gasto et al. physiological monitoring with accompanying EEG was performed during eye compression inducing periods of severe breath-holding in 24 subjects [94:1063-1067-c]. The groups were divided into children demonstrating strong cardiac inhibition (asystole) with little respiratory effect (pale group), intense respiratory inhibition and weak cardiac action (cyanotic group), and a third group demonstrating both cardiorespiratory inhibition (mixed group). In each group, at the onset of colour change, bradycardia and/or bradypnoea, the EEG demonstrated a burst of slow waves [96]. Similar results were subsequently demonstrated by a number of investigators [114:87-98-c]. This sequence was extended by Gauck et al. who recorded events in twenty children lasting up to 40 seconds, with clinical evolution occurring during full inspiratory exhalation [118:3130-3139-c]. They determined that cyanotic attacks develop during a series of four distinct phases: provocation, expiratory apnoea, rigidity and stupor [121:109-114-c].

"Prolonged exhalation apnea" with arterial hypertension is originally presented by Southall et al. in a physiological monitoring study involving 8 children, and was subsequently expanded to 51 children [30:155-160-c].

Researchers have studied the role of iron deficiency anaemia in the pathogenesis of ARP, but these results have been contradictory. J.Holowach et al. (1963) also noted that iron deficiency anaemia is frequently found in children with ARP, especially in patients with severe and frequent affective-respiratory paroxysms. M. Bhatia et al (1990) found that ARP was more common in socially disadvantaged families where the risk of iron deficiency in children was increased due to possible malnutrition. X. Genconul et al (2002) found evidence of iron deficiency anaemia in 60% of children with ARP. Decreased haemoglobin iron concentration was found to affect the frequency and severity of paroxysms. In addition, W. Franklin et al (1997) found a direct association between maternal iron deficiency anaemia and the incidence of ARP in infants [12:155-160-c]. Many studies that have reliably demonstrated the efficacy of treatment of children with ARP with iron-containing drugs suggest a possible pathogenetic relationship between iron deficiency anaemia in the child and the development of ARP. A positive effect, i.e., complete cessation or significant reduction in the frequency of paroxysms, was also observed in cases where anaemia was absent [21].

The role of iron deficiency in the development of ARP in children is unclear. It is believed that iron deficiency anaemia results in decreased oxygen saturation of the lungs, which leads to decreased oxygenation of body tissues, including the brain [30:155-161-c]. Metabolism of catecholamines in the body is impaired due to decreased iron concentration in the child, leading to impaired neurotransmitter and enzyme function in the central nervous system. Makan et al. (1999) studied the interaction of erythropoietin, nitric oxide and interleukin-1 in the brain to assess the role of iron deficiency anaemia in ARP. Treatment with iron-containing preparations increased erythropoietin concentration and reduced ARP attacks in children [14;63-c].

The strong association between anaemia and ARP was first reported in 1963 and has since been confirmed by others. It is estimated that between 23.5% and 69% of children with ARP are iron deficient, and many are anaemic. Clinical trials aimed at treating iron deficiency in patients with ARP have been conducted but have been limited by small sample sizes and inconsistent methodology [129].

Currently, much attention is paid to the "psychogenic-neurotic" factor in the development of ARP. But during the development of paroxysm it was found that, although the cause of the child's crying is involuntary, reflex movement, that is, the child consciously cannot bring himself into a state of apnoea, much less into a state of loss of consciousness. Neurotic children are more likely to have an increased incidence of ARP. However, from the point of view of some experts, treating the problem of ARP formation as "hysterical reactions of a young child" or "hysterical behaviour" is considered unacceptable and even more incorrect. Some studies did not increase the risk of behavioural and psycho-emotional disorders in such children compared to the control group.

The relationship between behavioural problems, emotional factors and breath-holding attacks has been discussed by many researchers. Breath-holding attacks have been described by by Abt [1918] as occurring in "neuropathic children of neuropathic parents". Bridge et al. [1943] found that children prone to breath-holding are usually of the active, energetic type, responding vigorously to situations, and that the episodes are provoked by "spoilt childish reactions". KKanner [1935] regarded breath-holding episodes as a sign of disturbed parent-child relationships. ЛакLaxdal et al. [1969]reported that 30 per cent of children with breath-holding episodes had abnormal behaviour, including angry outbursts, hyperactivity and stubbornness. To further investigate the role of behaviour and breath holding ДиМариDiMario and Burleson [1993] studied the behaviour of children with breath-holding episodes compared to controls and found no differences in behavioural profiles, suggesting that breath-holding episodes are involuntary and cannot be equated with a difficult child in temperament.

The relationship between ARP and emotions has long been a matter of debate. Some authors have observed that children with affective respiratory paroxysm have certain characteristic traits that make them prone to easily fall into despair and indecision [33;34-8-c]. If children with ARP have a difficult temperament, parents may need to adapt their parenting strategies to the child's temperament. These adapted parenting techniques may be helpful in shaping the difficult behaviours of these children, and this may reduce stress for parents.

N. Anas et al. (1991) found that laryngeal spasm occurs in young children due to local excitation of receptors in the upper part of the larynx caused by changes in the chemical composition of inhaled air, which can lead to prolonged respiratory arrest. Indirectly, A. Taylor et al. (1976) confirmed this possible mechanism, which proved the development of apnoea by mechanical irritation of the corresponding nerve in primate infants [72;203-8-c].

Thus, the main pathogenetic mechanisms of ARP development in young children are not yet fully understood, which becomes a trivial medical problem.

§1.3 Clinical manifestations of affective-respiratory paroxysms

Affective-respiratory seizures are a special type of anoxic seizures or syncope most commonly seen in young children in whom anoxic seizures or syncope are provoked, or precipitated, by a painful stimulus. Various provoking factors have been identified, but the most common is a sudden blow to the head.

After a painful physical or psychological experience, a child may briefly choke or cry and then lose consciousness. The child will collapse if they have been standing (Appleton, 1993; Martin et al, 2010) and appear very pale and lethargic. Parents often describe their child as dead pale, "looking as if he/she is dead" (Appleton, 1993; Blackmore, 1999). In addition, the child may become stiff (tonic) with twitching of limbs (clonic) (Meyer, 2009). An episode of ARP is usually brief, sometimes lasting less than 15 seconds, but can last up to a minute. Recovery is rapid and upward eye deviation as well as urinary incontinence has been reported (Appleton, 1993; Meyer, 2009: Tidy, 2012). Once conscious, the child may feel tired, exhausted and emotional for some time. This phase corresponds to a period of self-resolving asystole (Appleton, 1993; Meyer, 2009: Warrington, 2004; Tidy, 2012). Cases of prolonged unconsciousness are also known (Meyer, 2009). The cyanotic variant of ARP is characterised by the development of rapidly changing stages, which makes it possible to make the appropriate diagnosis at the time of history taking and to make a differential diagnosis with epileptic seizures and paroxysmal states.

Under the influence of unexpected emotionally provoking factors (fear, dissatisfaction, anger, painful stimulus, etc.), the child screams violently and starts crying, which lasts for more than 10-15 seconds.

At the peak of the cry, during the exhalation period, the child stops breathing (apnoea). At this time, the child's consciousness is impaired for a few seconds, but in this case the parents will be indifferent to the situation as a result of other distractions. The child has a diffuse decrease in muscle tone and the entire body is covered with a cyanotic tinge. The child takes a deep breath and regains consciousness - this is called an affective-respiratory paroxysm, depending on its clinical presentation. The duration of loss of consciousness at the end of an ARP attack is usually 20-60 seconds, in rare cases it may last longer. After this short period, the child's breathing, consciousness and motor activity recover quickly and spontaneously. The child often remains cranky after the seizure and continues to scream [41;353-355-c].

To date, there are no known cases of consecutive onset of several paroxysms in a row, i.e. a consecutive course of apnoea attacks seems to be an exclusion criterion for the diagnosis of ARP. Additional somatic disorders in the child, infectious diseases, fever, fatigue, emotional excitement of the child may lead to an increase in affective-respiratory attacks.

In some cases, the atypical course of ARP leads to certain diagnostic difficulties in the early stages. For example, the absence of clear anamnestic data on the presence of an initial provoking stimulus, in some cases the development of diffuse hypertonus instead of muscular hypotonia, sometimes the head is thrown back, and elements of opisthotonus are present. Paroxysm may be accompanied by twitching of individual muscles or even one limb. After the seizure, a short period of drowsiness or disorientation may be observed in the child [51;585-589-c].

Up to 15% of children with severe ARP experience a generalised anoxic epileptic seizure in the latter stages of the seizure, characterised by prolonged clonic jerks and a 'slow spike' on the EEG [33;34-38-c]. The paroxysm ends with a sudden gasp and a rapid return to consciousness, unless prolonged by an oxygen-free epileptic seizure [33;34-38-c].

Pale breath-holding episodes are more often provoked by pain or fear than by anger or frustration [88;354-361-c]. Episodes of pallor are less common than cyanotic episodes. Episodes of breath-holding are associated with the child crying for up to a minute and then not inhaling until he or she loses consciousness. A seizure may rarely occur immediately after loss of consciousness. The child usually regains consciousness soon afterwards and regains normal breathing. In both types, if the duration of unconsciousness exceeds approximately 45 seconds, tonic postures, opisthotonus, or clonic limb movements may be observed [12;155-160-c]. Although these seizures are inherently harmless, they can nevertheless cause fear and distress to parents. [12;155-160-c].

Affective-respiratory paroxysms in the child, regardless of when they occur, disappear at the age of 4-6 years and often much earlier. At present, ARP has no serious consequences, but some literature describes isolated exceptional observations and case descriptions resulting in sudden cardiac asystole and even death associated with "pale" ARP. In addition, D. Southall et al. (1990)

reported infant mortality with the "bluish" variant of ARP in 15% of cases, which has led to disbelief and criticism. It should be noted that [14;136-c] Palchik A. B. and Poniatishin A. E. (2012) noting in their study that they had no adverse findings associated with ARP based on more than 20 years of experience in the neurology department of an "emergency department".

It has been found that the risk of epilepsy, persistent neurological or significant intellectual impairment in children with ARP does not exceed the population average [21]. According to various reports, definitive development of epilepsy occurs in 0.5-11% of patients with ARP [87;127-151-c]. Syncope, especially in children with BARP, may develop later in 17% of adolescents [62;82-84-c].

In a population-based study conducted in Geelong, Australia (Geelong Study) from a population sample of 4988 people. Seventy-three children born in the early 1970s and followed from birth to 11 years of age developed severe ARF. This subgroup of children had a higher incidence of febrile seizures (9.6%) compared with children without ARP (5.2%), and a higher incidence of non-epileptic seizures (11% versus 3.2%) (51 of 73 were under complete follow-up) [29;171-183-c]. No other abnormal findings specific to this group were found.

Serious complications with afferent-respiratory paroxysms are rare. Taiwo and Hamilton [1993] reported a prolonged cardiac arrest in a patient with attacks of ARP. The few reported deaths may have been triggered by aspiration or occurred in children who were in severe respiratory arrest, often with structural airway abnormalities or a complicated history [Paulson, 1963 ; Southall et al, 1987 , 1990].

Several studies have shown that children with "cyanotic" ARP have a slightly increased risk of developing attention deficit hyperactivity disorder or behavioural disorders in old age compared with controls [91;496-498-c]. Children with the "pale" variant of ARP often experience syncopal states or other manifestations of transient autonomic dysfunction during adolescence or young adulthood [92;234-240-c].

Thus, the results of this study show that the clinical symptoms identified in children with ARP indicate the presence of a psychosomatic component in the genesis of this disease [15;61-65-c].

§1.4 Neurophysiological markers in the clinical assessment of newborns and infants

It is very important that practitioners collect a detailed and targeted history, as episodes of ARP can easily be misdiagnosed as epilepsy. Up to 50% of parent-reported seizure episodes, after careful history taking, were found to be thought to be related to anoxic seizures rather than epileptic events (Stephenson, 2001). In a study involving 380 children under the age of 16 who experienced "seizures, syncope", ARP was the main cause of non-epileptic seizures (Hindley et al., 2006). This has not changed much in recent years, in particular, overdiagnosis of epilepsy is increasing due to the active development of the epilepsy problem. Often symptoms of loss of consciousness, tonic and clonic muscle contractions, including urinary incontinence, may not be the reason for the diagnosis of epilepsy. A history of febrile seizures, enuresis, and sleep disturbances may not be sufficient factors in the diagnosis of epilepsy [29;171-183-c].

Diagnosis is usually made by a paediatrician on the basis of history. An ECG is usually performed at first episode as part of the initial baseline investigations to rule out cardiac arrhythmias, prolonged QT syndrome, cardiac AV blockade or ventricular hypertrophy. However, all of these conditions are extremely rare. An EEG (electroencephalogram) is also indicated as a baseline examination when ARP is suspected. Both ECG and EEG findings will be normal for ARP (Martin et al, 2010; Tide, 2012). The location of peak waves on the EEG on different leads should be carefully interpreted as they may be benign. For adequate evaluation of EEG is also of great importance the method of conducting the study taking into account the age and functional state of the child (Gorbacheva F.E., 2004.).

Nowadays, the diagnosis of epilepsy is very serious and it is necessary to know the diagnostic criteria and re-examine it over a period of time, as taking anticonvulsant drugs can lead to serious complications for the body. Non-epileptic paroxysms should be distinguished from generalised and partial epileptic seizures (Gorbacheva F.E., 2004.). Paediatric syncope, paroxysmal dyskinesia, parasomnia and pseudoepileptic (psychogenically induced) seizures are often mistaken as epileptic disorders. Loss of consciousness is also caused by acute transient cerebral ischaemia.

In some studies, changes in MRI and EEG signs have not been found in children with affective-respiratory paroxysms. In most cases, the diagnosis is made on the basis of clinical findings and history or home videos provided. Accordingly, EEG studies are not recommended for these children. Conventional EEG is sometimes necessary to reassure parents that the child has no epileptiform activity [29;171-183-c].

Neuroimaging studies such as computed tomography (CT) and magnetic resonance imaging (MRI) of the head are normal in children with breath-holding and are not necessary. Electroencephalography (EEG) is also usually not needed. Although the child may look like he or she has had a seizure, no seizures are seen on EEG in children during episodes. If a child has a shaking seizure that lasts more than two minutes, an EEG may be ordered because the child may be having a seizure caused by periods of breath-holding. The doctor may order blood tests to check for anaemia, as treating anaemia may reduce the frequency of breath-holding seizures. An electrocardiogram (ECG) may be ordered if symptoms do not match a typical episode of breath-holding (Sarah Roddy, 2020)

§1.5 Neurochemical mechanisms in the pathogenesis of affective-respiratory paroxysms

The nervous system is a morphologically and functionally very complex system, the main function of which is to regulate and control biochemical processes occurring in the human and animal body. This occurs mainly as a result of the peculiarities of the composition and metabolism of nervous tissue. Recently, there has been a significant increase in interest in the control of key brain functions using peptides. A fairly large number of peptides have been discovered which, in very low concentrations, can affect nervous tissue, acting as modulators of a number of functions as well as the actions of neurotransmitters, hormones and pharmacological agents. Peptides can in some cases modify behavioural responses, they are involved in memory mechanisms [16;74-76-c]. Given the preferred localisation of these peptides in the CNS, they have been termed neuropeptides (NPs). Small to medium-sized peptides are categorised as neuropeptides, ranging from 2 to 50-60 amino acid residues (a. o.). Hormones and a number of cell growth factors are categorised as large peptides [15;61-65-c]. NPs are formed by proteolysis of large peptides ("target"). These are synthesised in ribosomes and then transported to nerve terminal vesicles, cleaved by proteases to final forms of NPs and secreted to neurotransmitters [17;61-65-c].

Neuropeptides are synthesised not only in the hypothalamus but also in the brain and other parts of the body. By synthesising lyberin and statins, the hypothalamus stimulates the production of pituitary hormones and manifests itself by acting on certain neurons in the brain and other cells in the body. Thus, neuropeptides are powerful stimulators of emotional behaviour, motor activity, respiratory centre, etc.

In past centuries, melatonin was considered the most mysterious and ambiguous hormone. Melatonin is secreted by the pinealocyte cells of the vitreous at night from tryptophan to hydroxytryptophan and serotonin. Two enzymes, arylalkylamine-Nacetyltransferase (AA-NAT) and acetylserotonin-O-methyltransferase (ASMT), then form melatonin from serotonin [113;51-c]. The organisation of the sleep-wake rhythm in children occurs at about 6 months of age, but melatonin production in the healthy child begins at 3 months of age

The results of the study show that melatonin modulates the electrical activity of neurons in the brain. Melatonin has the property to affect GABAergic, 5NT-ergic and NO/L-arginine pathways and mediates glutamate neurotransmission [115; 648-652-c]. Research studies by Ross et al, 2018 revealed the antioxidant and neurometabolic property of melatonin in children with epilepsy. Stewart and Lyon (2021) suggest that the proconvulsive effects of melatonin inhibit GAMK A receptors in pyramidal cells. In 2005, Hancock et al in a further randomised double-blind crossover study determined that administration of melatonin (5 mg) in the treatment of epilepsy in 31 patients aged 8 months to 18 years resulted in a reduction in seizure frequency. During a conference in Rome in 2014, Bruni et al. gave instructions and recommendations for melatonin treatment of children with neurodevelopmental disorders.

Sleep problems in children with delayed psychomotor development may be associated with impaired melatonin secretion and decreased sensitivity of melatonin receptors. Generally, sleep disorders are the most common problems in the paediatric population. The prevalence of sleep problems in childhood is observed between 30 and 40% [112; 2012-2023-c]. Sleep deprivation at the cellular level increases oxidative stress in the hippocampus and contributes to the loss of synaptic circuitry of neurons, which may affect neurocognitive disorders, especially attention, behavioural and emotional developmental aspects (Justyna Paprocka, 2018).

In the last decade, melatonin has been considered as an optimal option to minimise neurological complications of hypoxic-ischaemic nervous system injury [113;51-c]. Due to the extreme sensitivity of the brain to peroxidation products, free oxygen radicals, oxidative stress develops (Stewart LS, 2005;46:473-480). This process is regulated by the lipid composition of biomembranes and is also involved in the synthesis of leukotrienes, prostaglandins, catecholamine metabolism and affects the ability of membranes to permeate and transport substances across them [95;1010-105-c]. The most popular methods to assess lipid peroxidation are the determination of oxidation products of polyunsaturated fatty acids: levels of malonic dialdehyde (MDA) and conjugated dienes (DC). Diene conjugates (DCs) are toxic metabolites that damage proteins, enzymes and nucleic acids [94; 393-399-c].

Melatonin may serve as a potential therapeutic free radical scavenger (hydroxyl radicals, hydrogen peroxide, singlet oxygen) and a broad-spectrum antioxidant (activation of antioxidant pathways; superoxide dismutase, catalase, glutathione peroxidase, glutathione reductase) [119;51-c].

Children after hypoxic-ischaemic brain damage often develop circadian rhythm disturbances. Studies by Yang et al. proved melatonin secretion from epithelial cells is impaired after hypoxic nervous system injury [119;51-c]. They suggested that miR-325-3p (microRNA) may play a role as a potential down-regulator of the

AANAT rate-limiting enzyme for melatonin synthesis (Justyna Paprocka, 2018).

Antioxidant activity of melatonin

Melatonin is produced in the pineal gland, retina and possibly in some other organs. Melatonin's functions as an antioxidant include; a) direct scavenging of free radicals, b) stimulation of antioxidant enzymes, c) increasing the efficiency of mitochondrial oxidative phosphorylation (thereby reducing free radical formation) and d) increasing the efficiency of other antioxidants. There may be other functions of melatonin, as yet undiscovered, that enhance its ability to protect against molecular damage by oxygen- and nitrogen-based toxic reagents. Numerous studies have confirmed the ability of both physiological and pharmacological concentrations of melatonin to protect against free radical damage [83;5-22-c].

In modern medicine, some studies have used melatonin in many cases to reduce oxidative stress. This has been achieved in various ways; by direct neutralisation of reactive oxygen species and reactive nitrogen species and indirect stimulation of antioxidant enzymes, while inhibiting the activity of oxidative enzymes.

The results show that melatonin and its metabolites have potent antioxidant and anti-inflammatory effects that protect mainly nuclear and mitochondrial DNA in all cells [86;151-180-c].

Its antioxidant action is believed to be much stronger than that of vitamins E and C and glutathione. The molecule can capture up to 10 AFCs (reactive oxygen species) compared to classical antioxidants, which neutralise one or fewer AFCs (9). The protective effect of melatonin is to increase the activity of antioxidant enzymes including superoxide dismutase (SOD), catalase (K), and glutathione peroxidase (GPO) by increasing the expression of the aforementioned enzymes (75;1-9-c). In addition, melatonin is located on the surface of cell membranes near the polar heads of phospholipids, consequently protecting cell membranes from oxidation. By altering the fluidity of membranes, it removes radicals before they damage the lipids and proteins of the cell membrane. Melatonin has no pro-oxidant properties [75;1-9-c].

Melatonin acts as a free radical scavenger and as an indirect antioxidant. It scavenges hydroxyl radicals produced by the Fenton reaction and reduces lipid peroxidation in the brain, as well as blocking toxicity caused by singlet oxygen. Studies on rats with induced stroke and removed pineal glands showed that administration of melatonin at a dose of 5 mg kg-1 at the onset of reperfusion resulted in improvement in the animals. A reduction in ischaemic areas in the grey matter and white brain was observed, as well as a reduction in the inflammatory response, and brain oedema was reduced. In addition, modern studies show the protective effect of melatonin on glial cells [86;151-180-c].

Venkataraman et al (2020) study results showed that melatonin significantly reduces neuronal damage during oxidative stress induced by exposure to neurotoxins by increasing the activity of antioxidant enzymes such as total superoxide dismutase (TSSD) and glutathione peroxidase (GPO). As mentioned earlier, melatonin was found to cause a decrease in total peroxidation and malonic aldehyde [109;189-197-c].

Thus, the antioxidant action of melatonin is based on its direct and indirect induction of antioxidant enzymes. It has been shown that these mechanisms of melatonin action are associated with its oncostatic, immunomodulatory, rejuvenating and neuroprotective effects.

The aforementioned effect of melatonin would indicate that it is one of the most powerful antioxidants.

Conclusions to Chapter I;

Non-epileptic paroxysmal conditions of childhood are a group of disorders, syndromes and phenomena that mimic true epileptic seizures. They span ages from newborn to young adult and may be the most common diagnostic problems clinicians encounter on a regular basis. The key to diagnosis is a detailed history and careful observation.

Detection of "non-epileptic paroxysmal conditions" helps clinicians avoid unnecessary and potentially inappropriate treatment and reduces the risk of epilepsy. Longitudinal monitoring and re-evaluation are important aspects of diagnostic accuracy.

One of the most frequently observed non-epileptic paroxysmal states in young children is affective-respiratory paroxysms (ARP), manifested by involuntary breath-holding with short-term impairment of consciousness and motor activity on exogenous stimuli. In modern practice, ARP leads to misdiagnosis of epilepsy due to similar paroxysmal conditions (loss of consciousness, apnoea, cyanosis, sometimes the presence of tonic and convulsive spasms).

The development of ARP may result from congenital transient dysfunction (dysregulation) of the child's autonomic nervous system, associated somatic diseases (anaemia, hypocalcaemia) and increased sensitivity and susceptibility to respiratory spasms in young children due to changes in the chemical composition of exhaled air.

Brain hypoxia, imbalance of the antioxidant system, and increased oxidative stress play a role in the pathogenesis of ARP development. Scientists in their studies have suggested that melatonin reduces the formation of the destructively toxic hydroxyl radical, which leads to a decrease in oxidative stress. The prevalence of melatonin in all tissues, including its high concentration in mitochondria, likely contributes to its ability to resist oxidative stress and apoptosis. There is strong evidence that melatonin should be noted as a mitochondria-targeted antioxidant. The ability of melatonin to prevent oxidative damage (ischaemia/reperfusion, hypoxia/reoxygenation) especially in the brain (stroke) and heart (heart attack) and related diseases is well demonstrated in many experimental studies. Due to its antiradical mechanisms, melatonin has been found in studies to reduce drug toxicity. Experimental evidence suggests that melatonin delays the development of various age-related diseases and may be useful for treatment.

In connection with the above, the identification of risk factors for the development of ARP and the study of clinical, neurological, and neurophysiological characteristics improve treatment tactics and prevent the development of epilepsy.

CHAPTER II. MATERIAL AND METHODS OF RESEARCH CHILDREN WITH ARP

§2.1 General characteristics of the examined patients

Based on the objectives of the study, a clinical examination of 103 patients of children with affective-respiratory paroxysms at the age of three months to three years was carried out. All patients underwent inpatient and outpatient treatment in the clinic of the Tashkent Paediatric Medical Institute in 2019-2022.

Children were included in the main group according to the following criteria; children under 3 years of age, paroxysmal disorders of consciousness, presence of non-epileptic seizure, parental consent for continued examination and psychological test.

The following criteria were not included in the survey; congenital brain defects; inherited metabolic disorders (cystic fibrosis), chromosomal and autoimmune diseases.

The control group consisted of 20 "conditionally healthy" children. Children in the control group were examined by a paediatrician as part of a standard check-up during the outpatient follow-up period.

The necessary conditions for inclusion of children in the control group are absence of delayed physical and psychomotor development of the child (PMD), absence of registration with a neurologist with neurological diseases in the first year of life, successful pregnancy and labour history, satisfactory condition at birth, Apgar score of the child should be at least 7-9 points, neuropsychiatric condition and physical development should correspond to the age and during the examination parents should not complain about pathology of the nervous system

The age characteristics were comparable in the compared groups. The mean age of the main group of children was 13.3 ± 7.2 months, in the control group 20.9 ± 6.4 months, of which 54 children under 12 months of age; 30 children under 13-24 months of age; and 19 children under 25-36 months of age. In the main group, boys 69 (66.9%) predominated over girls 34 (33.0%) (sex ratio 2:1).

The age distribution of children in the compared groups is shown in Table 2.1. (Table 2.1.).

Table 2.1.

Distribution of examined patients by age and sex

Age	Paul			
	Main group n=103		Control group n=20	
	Boys	Girls	Boys	Girls
3-12 months	34	20	8	4
13-24 months	21	9	1	2
25-36 months	14	5	3	2
Bottom line:	69	34	12	8

§2.2 Clinical, laboratory and instrumental methods of investigation

The study examined in detail the history data of each child, irrespective of their group, and also analysed in detail the hereditary, family and social history given by the parents and relatives of the patients.

We divided *risk factors* into 3 subgroups to assess the impact on the development of ARP: 1) data of obstetric and gynaecological history; 2) data of neonatal period; 3) sociobiological factors;

A neurological examination was performed sequentially, assessing the state of higher brain functions, cranial nerves, motor sphere (voluntary movements, coordination, involuntary movements), sensitive sphere, meningeal syndromes and autonomic-trophic functions.

When assessing the neurological status of the child, symptoms of intracranial hypertension, motor activity, pyramidal signs, muscle tone, tendon reflexes, newborn reflexes, behavioural abnormalities, disorders of physical and psychomotor development of the child (PMD), sleep disorders, regurgitation, unreasonable restlessness, anxiety, and meteorological dependence were taken into account.

In the research work, we evaluated the state of the nervous system of children under 1 year of age using the classification of complications of central nervous system lesions in the perinatal period, created by N.N. Volodin, A.S. Petrukhin (2009).

To assess the psychomotor development of children, we used the method of Pantyukhin G.V., Pechora K.L., Frucht E.L. (2007) [18]. The methodology is a qualitative assessment of child development without the use of points. The table gives indicators of development of children from 10 days to 3 years of life (norm) on the main lines of development (speech comprehension, active speech, sensory development, play, movements, skills, constructive activity, visual activity and behaviour).

The methodology determines the formation of the first visual and auditory reactions of newborns. In the period from the end of the neonatal period to 5-6 months of age, such indicators as the development of visual and auditory reactions, emotions, contact between children and parents, fine motor skills, large motor skills and active speech are tested. From 6 to 12 months of age, the development of joint actions, movement with objects, understanding of active speech, children's relationships with each other, and emotional development are assessed.

In Year 2, speech comprehension, active speech, emotional development, movement and skills, and play activity are diagnosed.

In the 3rd year of life, speech comprehension, active speech, attitudes towards games, skills in constructive and visual activities, and emotional development behaviour are tested (Table 2.2.1.).

Table 2.2.1.

Indicators of neuropsychological development of children under three years of age

Age	*Level of neuropsychological development*								Behaviour	Conclusion (epicr.cf.)
	Understanding speeches	Active speech	Touch development	Game	movements	Skills	Constructive activity	Pictorial activity		

In the 1st year of life, the psychomotor development of the child is normal for the formation of skills within +15 days of the normal accepted age indicated in the table. In the 2nd year of life - within a quarter, in the 3rd year of life - half a year. Based on the established norm, skill formation 1 epicrisis period earlier indicates early development, and skill formation 2 or more epicrisis periods earlier indicates rapid development. A 1 epicrisis period delay in skill acquisition indicates a slow rate of development. To quantify the neuropsychological development of children, K.L. Pechora developed a method that assesses the depth and range of delay in children. For this purpose, 5 groups of developers were identified [18]. The 1st group of children with normal development. Children are included in the 2nd group if they are developmentally delayed by 1 epicrisis term. Children are included in group 3 if they are developmentally delayed for 2 epicrisal periods. Children are included in Group 4 if they are developmentally delayed for 3 epicrisal periods. Children are included in group 4 if they are behind in development for 3 epicrisis periods, i.e. 9 months delay. Children are included in group 5 if they are 4 epicrisis periods behind in development.

The study of the vegetative status of the child also has prognostic potential in many clinical situations. Analysis of the state of the autonomic nervous system is of great importance for the diagnosis of ARP.

The ANS is an integral part of the nervous system and is responsible for controlling vital functions such as heartbeat, breathing and digestion. It is also involved in the response to stress. The presence of underlying autonomic nervous system dysfunction in children with ARP has been suggested by many authors.

In the differential diagnosis of epilepsy with syncope, it is important to identify autonomic dysfunction. Several dominant forms of episodes may be observed in ARP patients, i.e. cyanotic, pale and mixed seizures may occur simultaneously, but the activity of the autonomic nervous system is of great importance in their manifestation. Since there are differences in the clinical manifestations of ARP in children, we will consider these groups separately, but recognise that they have partial similarities.

To analyse the state and regulatory capacity of the autonomic nervous system, an excellent and meaningful tool at our disposal is: baseline autonomic tone, autonomic support and reactivity. Autonomic disorders in children can be generalised or systemic.

Unlike adults, panic disorders in children have their own peculiarities depending on the age of the child. There is a predominance of vegetative-somatic manifestations in the attack structure over panic and emotional experiences in younger children.

In older age groups, the vagus orientation of reactions decreases, the sympathetic component in paroxysms increases, which reflects the general intensification of humoral regulatory connection.

The initial vegetative tone was assessed using an adapted table for children developed by A.M. Vein et al. (1998) from the Department of Paediatrics of the Russian Medical Academy.

Table 2.2.2.

Table of A.M. Vein et al. (1998) for determining the initial vegetative tone of the organism.

Признак	Симпатикотония	Ваготония
Цвет кожи	Бледный	Склонность к покраснению
Сосудистый рисунок	Не выражен	Мраморность, акроцианоз
Сальность кожи	Снижена	повышена
Потоотделение	Уменьшена	повышено
Дермографизм	Розовый, белый	красный
Зябкость	Отсутствует	характерна
Температура при инфекциях	Склонность к гипертермии	Склонность к субфебрилитету
Переносимость душных помещении	Удовлетворительная	Плохая
Обмороки	Редко	Характерны
Головокружения	Не характерны	Характерны
Аппетит	Повышен	Может быт снижен
Масса тела	Склонность к похуданию	Может быт склонность к полноте
Число сердечных сокращений	Склонность к тахикардии	Склонность к брадикардии
Артериальное давление	Склонность к повышению	Склонность к понижению
Одышка	Не характерны	Характерны
Склонность к тошноте, рвоте, болям животе	Не характерна	Возможна
Боли в ногах по вечерам	Не характерны	Могут быть
Головные боли	бывают	частые
Сон	беспокойный	Глубокий, продолжительный

The sum of vagotonic and sympathicotonic signs is calculated from this table. If the number of vagotonic signs does not exceed four and the number of sympathicotonic signs does not exceed two, this condition is called eutonia. If the number of points in any system exceeds six, it indicates an increase in the autonomic tone of this system.

To determine the functional reserve of adaptation of children taking into account age features, a passive orthostatic test (telt test, Kenny 1986) was carried out, with the child's head raised to a height of 30 degrees.

General clinical examination was carried out in the standard way: the state of the musculoskeletal system, respiratory organs, cardiovascular, gastrointestinal and genitourinary systems were examined in turn to identify somatic pathology and comorbid background. Children of the main group were thoroughly examined by narrow specialists - paediatrician, ophthalmologist, otolaryngologist, orthopaedist, paediatric surgeon and cardiologist, etc., if somatic disorders were identified.

Laboratory methods of investigation included:

1. general haematological and biochemical blood tests;

2. serum content of biochemical markers (malonic dialdehyde (MDA) and diene conjugates (DC), superoxide dismutase (SOD), glutathione peroxidase, glutathione reductase, catalase, cytochrome C-oxidase and nitric oxide (NO)) was determined by spectrophotometric method;

Peripheral (venous) blood sera were used as a substrate for determination of AOS and POL markers.

Neuroimaging was performed using transcranial ultrasound tomography. In our research work, we used a SONIX scanner

(Canada, 2007) consisting of a 5-2 MGS sector transducer and a 14-15 MGS linear transducer. Ultrasonography was performed using standard methods, when the patient was hospitalised, data were recorded and compared with previous data. Ultrasound examination of other organs was performed when indicated.

Neurophysiological *examination* included electroencephalography (EEG). EEG registration was performed on a 16-channel electroencephalograph "Neurocartograph-1-MBN" of the scientific and medical firm "MVN" (manufactured in 2003).

The "paper movement" speed was 30 mm/sec. The calibration signal was 50 mV, the amplitude was 50 mW, the value of the high-pass filters was 30 Hz, the sensitivity of the valves was 50 μV, and the resistance of the electrodes was not higher than 10 kOhm. The research work was carried out in a dark, quiet room in a special chair or in the mother's arms. EEG results were obtained mainly in the morning in physiological sleep state, sometimes in waking state. Sleep was monitored by behavioural criteria (prolonged eye closure) and autonomic indices (decreased heart rate and muscle tone). Monopolar recording was performed using the Nero programme. The method and procedure for placing electrodes on the child's head coincided with the international standard scheme.

§2.3 Biochemical methods of research

The following markers were selected to assess the role of lipid peroxidation and antioxidant system in the development of affective-respiratory paroxysms in children (Table 2.3.1.):

Table 2.3.1.

Biochemical markers investigated

POL indicators analysed				
malonic dialdehyde		dienketones		
AOH enzymes				
Superoxide dismutase (SOD)	Catalase	Glutathione reductase	Glutathione peroxidase	Glutathione -S-transferase
Protein				
Nitrous oxide				
Cytochrome c oxidase				

For the research work, venous blood (3-5 ml) was collected under sterile conditions in the procedure room using Vasuette and Greiner bio-opaque tubes (manufactured in Austria).

Then "standard centrifugation procedure (Nimac CT 6E/CT 6EL machine) was performed to obtain serum (determination of biochemical parameters and assessment of antioxidant status) and citrate plasma (determination of general blood count and thiol groups)" (Koleschenko P.D. 2012). (Kolesnichenko P. D., 2012).

Lipids are molecules that are sensitive to oxygen due to their molecular structure with a large number of double hydrogen bonds. Free radicals initiate and cause lipid peroxidation, especially in cell membranes, and are associated with various pathophysiological changes, mainly vascular damage. Lipid peroxidation can have various effects on cellular functions, either directly, by reacting with proteins and nucleic acids, or indirectly, through receptor signalling pathways. Thus, lipid peroxidation of membrane lipids leads to changes in blood flow, increased permeability and decreased membrane potential2, which can lead to cell death. Among aldehydes from secondary products of lipid peroxidation, the most important are malonic dialdehyde (MDA), diene conjugates (DC), etc. (Table 2.3.2.) [24:223-233-c]. Since MDA has been one of the most popular and reliable markers for detecting oxidative stress in clinical practice for many years, it has been widely used in biomedical research as a biomarker [24:223-233-c].

Table 2.3.2.

Порядок внесения реагентов в пробу (мл)

Реагент	Опытная проба	Контрольная проба
Физиологический раствор	0,8	0,8
Дистиллированная вода	-	0,2
Плазма крови	0,2	-
ТХУ	0,5	0,5
Центрифугировали 15 мин при 1700г, отбирали супернатант		
Супернатант	1,0	1,0
ЭДТА	0,075	0,075
ТБК	0,25	0,25
Содержимое пробирок перемешивали и ставили в кипящую водяную баню на 15 мин. Затем пробирки охлаждали до комнатной температуры		

2.5 ml of citrated blood was placed in a centrifuge tube with a 10% solution of 2.5 ml trichloroacetic acid (TCA) and mixed thoroughly with a glass rod. The samples were centrifuged at 3000 rpm for 15 minutes. The precipitate was taken from 3.0 ml of the upper liquid and placed in a clean centrifuge tube, 1.5 ml of 0.8% 2-thiobarbituric acid was added and mixed thoroughly. The sample was placed in a boiling water bath for 15 minutes (Khamnagdaeva N.V., 2017).

Samples were taken from a boiling water bath and cooled in a stream of tap water. After cooling, they were 3000 rpm. When centrifuged for 15 min. Simultaneously with the experiments, control samples with 2.5 ml of 10% TCUK solution, 1.5 ml of 0.8% 2-thiobarbituric acid solution were also added. The resulting centrifuge tube is carefully placed in a chemical tube without spotting, and the control is 532 nm relative to the sample.at measured the optical density of the experimental samples. Calculation of results The amount of MDA is calculated based on the following formula. C=(E*10^6*3)/(1,56*10^5)

Methodological provisions for the study of free-radical oxidation processes and antioxidant defence system of the organism. Method of determination of malonic dialdehyde in blood. Voronezh. 2020. C. 37-39.

Determination of the content of diene conjugates. The method is based on the determination of the content of lipid peroxidation products in blood by absorption of ultraviolet light spectrum of lipid extract in the erythrocyte membrane by a stream of chromatic light. The amount of diene conjugates (DC) is extracted in heptane-isopropanol fractions.

Reagents:

1. n-heptane
2. isopropanal
3. 0.01 N aqueous hydrochloric acid solution
4. Calcined sodium chloride

Procedure: 8 ml of heptane-isopropanol was added to 0.1 ml of blood plasma, shaken for 15 minutes and centrifuged at 6000 rpm for

10 minutes. The lipid extract was then transferred into a clean test tube and 5 ml of heptane-isopropanol was added at a ratio of 3:7, 2 ml of 0.01 n aqueous chloride solution was added (Ivanovna, 2017).. The heptane phase was carefully withdrawn and used for further analysis. In order to remove water and water-soluble compounds from the lower aqueous-alcohol phase, 1.5g NaCl was added and shaken vigorously. The resulting lipids were dissolved in 5 ml of heptane-isopropanol (1:1) mixture and spectrophotometrically analysed. 232 nm (DK absorbance) was evaluated relative to the corresponding control at wavelengths.

Determination of catalase activity. Catalase protects the body from the toxic effects of hydrogen, which is formed under the influence of biological oxidation in tissues. The enzyme catalase in blood has a very high catalytic activity, which is considered to be heminferent. Colour intensity is measured at a wavelength of 410 nm against a sample that contains 2 ml of H_2 O instead of H O_{22} on a spectrophotometer (Table 2.3.3.).

Table 2.3.3.

	Контроль	Опыт	Премичание
H_2O_2	2 мл	2 мл	-
Сыворотки крови или гомогенат	-	0,1 мл	10 мин 37^{0}C
H_2O	0,1	-	
$(NH_4)_6Mo_7O_{24}$	1 мл	1 мл	-

The catalase activity in serum and tissues was expressed by the amount of catalase and calculated using the following formula.

$$(mcat/l)E=(A_{К\ oncontrol} - A_{опыт})*V*t*22.2$$

Korolyuk MA, Ivanova LI, Mayorova IG, Tokarev VE. Methods for determining the activity of catalase // Moscow., *Medicine*, 1988. C.16-18.

Determination of superoxide dismutase (SOD) enzyme activity. Determination of SOD enzyme activity (KF 1.15.1.1.1) by Misra and J. Fridovich (1972). was carried out according to the method. The principle of the method was formed as a result of aerobic interaction and NADH based on nitrotetrazol blue (NTS) for superoxide anions that block the amount of phenazymethasulphate (Table 2.3.4).

	Контроль	Опыт	Примечание
ТРИС-ЭДТА буфер. pH=7.4	0.05 мл	-	
Сыворотки крови или гомогенат	-	0.05 мл	
Реагент 1	2.0 мл	2.0 мл	10 минут 37^{0}C
Реагент 2	0.1 мл	0.1 мл	5 минут 25^{0}C

As a result of this reaction, NTS forms hydrozintetrazolium. In the presence of SOD, the percentage of NTS reduction decreases. The activity of NTS as a result of incubation of 50% of the enzyme reduction reaction is shown in units corresponding to 1 g of protein. The essence of the method is based on the reduction of nitrotetrazolium by blue and alkaline medium.

Matyushin B.N. Determination of superoxide dismutase activity in the material of puncture biopsy of the liver in its chronic lesions // Lab. *aff.* 1991. №7. C. 16-19.

Determination of glutathione reductase enzyme activity. In the determination of glutathione reductase (GR) activity (KF 1.6.4.2), the blood sample taken is centrifuged at 3000 rpm for 15 minutes, placed in sodium citrate at a ratio of 10:1, serum is removed and washed with physical solution. NADPH enzyme activity at 370°C is expressed at 1 minute in 1 g protein, micromole of NADPH compared to the decrease in NADPH at 340 nm wavelength for 10 minutes.

Vlasova SN, Shabunina EI, Pereslegina IA Activity of glutathione-dependent erythrocytes in chronic diseases. // Moscow. *Medicine,* 1990. C. 19-21.

Determination of glutathione peroxidase enzyme activity. Glutathione peroxidase is determined by the accumulation of oxidative glutathione: this occurs with the disappearance of oxidised glutathione and is detected at a wavelength of 260 nm. The activity of the enzyme is shown in μmol of glutathione in acid per 1 ha ha of haemoglobin.

Vlasova SN, Shabunina EI, Pereslegina IA Activity of glutathione-dependent erythrocytes in chronic diseases. // Moscow. *Medicine,* 1990. C. 19-21.

Determination of glutathione transferase enzyme activity. The reaction proceeds according to the following mechanism. The enzyme activity is determined by substrate 1-chloro, 2,4-dinitrobenzene.

glutathione + 1-chloro, 2,4-dinitrobenzene → glutathione-dinitrobenzene + HCl GT activity is determined at a wavelength of 340 nm.

Vlasova SN, Shabunina EI, Pereslegina IA Activity of glutathione-dependent erythrocytes in chronic diseases. // Moscow. *Medicine,* 1990. C. 19-21.

Determination of protein level. The amount of protein was determined using the Lowry method.

Lowry O.H., Rosenbrouch H.G., Farr A.L., Randall R., Protein measurement with the folin phenol reagent, *J. Biol. Chem.,* 1975, v. 193, no. 1.- P. 265-275.

Determination of cytochrome-C oxidase in serum.

Cytochrome-C oxidase (CsO) is a useful endogenous metabolic marker for neurons because the nervous system is highly dependent on aerobic metabolism for energy supply, and cytochrome oxidase plays an important role in mitochondrial aerobic energy metabolism (Wong-Riley 1989). Cytochrome-C oxidase levels were determined by enzyme immunoassay in serum samples using a commercial enzyme immunoassay kit (Human Caspase 8 Platinum ELISA) from eBioscience Inc according to the manufacturer's instructions. Threshold values of cytochrome-C oxidase determination in serum are 0.05ng/ml.

M Wikstrom, K Krab and M Saraste, Cytochrome Oxidase A Synthesis, Academic Press, London, 1981.

Determination of nitric oxide in plasma

Nitric oxide (NO), an endogenously generated gas, modulates the activity of CsO. At higher oxygen concentrations, when CsO is predominantly in the oxidised state, it consumes NO. At lower oxygen concentrations, when CsO is predominantly reduced, NO is not consumed and accumulates in the cell cavity, resulting in increased local vascular tone. Changes in intracellular oxygen concentration cause an increase in reactive oxygen species, leading to hypoxia in cells.

Procedure: Samples are deproteinised by adding 0.4 ml of methanol-diethyl ether (3:1) to 0.2 ml of plasma (serum) followed by centrifugation at 10000 rpm for 30 minutes. To 200 μl of the supernatant, 200 μl of saturated VCl3 solution is added. This intermediate is then allowed to react with the combination reagent, N-naphthyl ethylenediamine (NED), to form a stable azo compound. The overall reaction is described in the scheme below. The intense purple colour of the product allows nitrite analysis with high sensitivity and can be used to measure nitrite concentration at ~0.5

μM. The absorbance of this adduct at 540 nm is linearly proportional to the nitrite concentration in the sample. Because of the two-step nature of the Griess reaction, variations exist among published analyses of the Griess reaction. For example, CA and NED can be premixed in an acidic medium prior to interaction with nitrite. In yet another variation, after nitrite reacts with CA in acidic medium, NED is added after 10 minutes. The most popular variant is the sequential method, where nitrite is mixed with SA first and then NED is added immediately. (Figure 3.3.1.).

Kobylansky, T.V. Kuznetsova, G.N. Soboleva, O.N. Bondarenko, O.A. Pogorelova, V.N. Titov, V.P. Masenko. Pogorelova, V.N. Titov, V.P. Masenko. Nitric oxide determination in human serum and plasma by high-performance liquid chromotography. Biomedical Chemistry, 2003, Vol. 49 No. 6, pp. 597-603.

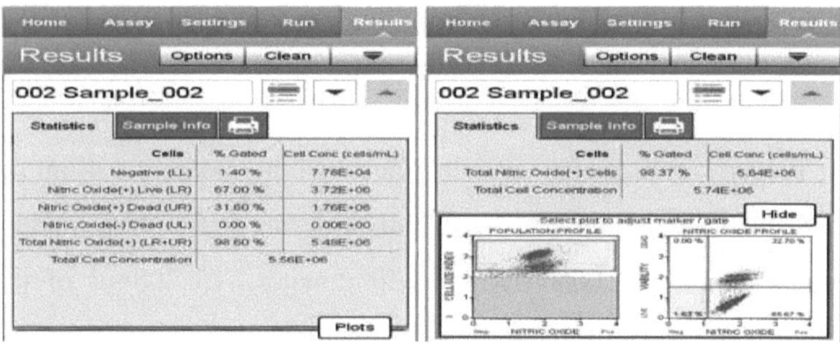

Figure 3.3.1: Nitric oxide *NOx* metabolites content in plasma of healthy children and patients (μmol/l).

§2.4 Treatment methods used

The treatment of affective-respiratory paroxysms requires differentiated and individualised treatment. The main goal of treatment of ARP is to relieve seizures and prevent transformation into epilepsy. The choice of therapy for patients with affective-respiratory paroxysms should be based on the presence of premorbid conditions, the nature of ARP attacks, the clinical and neurological status, the degree of severity of psychoemotional and behavioural symptoms, biochemical parameters, as well as the nature of neurophysiological parameters.

In order to substantiate pathogenetic therapy for the correction of ARP in children, we formed two main directions of therapy: pathogenetic and traditional (therapy according to clinical recommendations).

This principle of therapy was applied in all age groups.

- Pathogenetic therapy:

Scheme A: standard nootropic therapy + iron-containing drugs + melatonin;

- Conventional therapy:

Scheme B: standard nootropic therapy.

Children from Scheme A group (35 boys and 25 girls, mean age 13.7±5.6 months) were treated with melatonin combination therapy (Melglis drops in 50ml vials, SYNERGY GLOBAL IMPEX (PVT) LTD, Pakistan) once a day (2 hours before sleep) for 1 month. Children from 6 months to 1 year of age were given melatonin at a dose of 0.5 mg/day (3 drops), and from 1 to 3 years of age were given 1.0 mg/day (5 drops).

Patients from Scheme B group (25 boys and 9 girls, mean age 10.3±6.1 months) were treated with standard nootropic therapy only. As nootropic therapy we used the drug Noofen. The duration of treatment with Noofen was 4 weeks on average. The efficacy of treatment was evaluated on the basis of clinical and laboratory observations. Patients underwent extensive clinical, neurological and laboratory examination. Noofen dosage - up to 1 year of age was prescribed 50 mg once a day, *up* to 2 years of age 50 mg 2 times a day, children up to 3 years of age 100 mg 2 times a day.

Iron-containing preparations were administered to correct iron deficiency anaemia.

One month after treatment, biochemical parameters ((malonic dialdehyde (MDA) and diene conjugates (DC), superoxide dismutase (SOD), glutathione peroxidase, glutathione reductase, catalase, cytochrome-C oxidase and nitric oxide (NO)) in serum, frequency characteristics of paroxysms, severity of psychoemotional manifestations and indices of brain bioelectrical activity.

The efficacy of melatonin as an antioxidant agent has been confirmed in adults; however, its efficacy in paediatric practice is unclear.

§2.5 Statistical processing of the results obtained

The results of the study were carried out on optical measurements of a Cary 60 Agilent technology spectrophotometer. The obtained results were performed using Origin 6.1 (USA) computer programme for statistical processing and rendering of images. In the studies, the experimental model was carried out by the method of calculating the arithmetic mean value based on blood tests. The difference between the values obtained in the in vitro studies was calculated by t-criterion. In this case, $p<0.05$; $p<0.01$; values expressed the degree of statistical significance.

CHAPTER III. ANALYSIS OF ETIOPATHOGENETIC FACTORS IN THE DEVELOPMENT OF ARP

§3.1 Analysis of risk factors for affective-respiratory paroxysms in children

To achieve the objectives of the research work, 103 children with ARP were examined. They were distributed by gender as follows: 66.9% of boys and 33.0% of girls.

Within the framework of the study, an "Individual Patient Card" was developed, containing a retrospective clinical part (including antenatal period, newborn period, information on preventive vaccinations, diseases suffered and social history) and a prospective clinical part for the assessment and study of risk factors for the development of the disease in children, as well as the clinical picture of the disease.

A detailed study of obstetric and gynaecological history, neonatal data and socio-biological factors influencing the development of ARP was performed.

When analysing the data of obstetric and gynaecological anamnesis, pregnancy in women in 85.4% of cases was accompanied by genital and extragenital pathology. The most common pathologies were iron deficiency anaemia during pregnancy (85.4%), toxicosis during pregnancy (56.3%), risk of pregnancy termination (25.2%), pathological course of pregnancy (44.6%), spontaneous abortion in the history (34.9%), infectious and inflammatory diseases of the mother during pregnancy (28.1%), cardiovascular disease of the mother (7.8%) and exacerbation of chronic nasopharyngeal infection

(14.5%). Percentage study of obstetric and gynaecological history in the study shows that perfect pregnancy and delivery were very rare. The analysis of obstetric and gynaecological history data in the study is presented in Table 3.1.1.

Table 3.1.1.

Характеристика перинатального периода детей обеих групп

Показатель	I группа n (%)	II группа n (%)
Беременность по счету		
1	56,3	75
2	24,3	25
3	16,5	-
4	4,9	-
Прерывания беременности в анамнезе	34,9	10
Патология беременности (раннего и позднего гестоза)	44,6	5
Токсикозы беременности	56,3	20
Угрозы прерывания беременности	25,2	10
Инфекционные заболевания матери во время беременности	28,1	10
Цитомегаловирус	6,8	-
Вирус простого герпеса лаб/генит (обострение)	5,8	-
Хронический вирусный гепатит В	1,9	-
сердечно-сосудистые заболевания матери	7,8	-
Обострение хронической инфекции носоглотки (стрепт, стаф)	14,5	5
Анемия	85,4	20

When analysing the birth status of the studied children using individual medical records, the following clinical cases were identified: 44 (42.7%) children were born in satisfactory condition, 51 (49.5%) children were born in moderate condition and 5 (4.9%) children were born in severe condition. When analysing the gestational age of the children, the following was found: 73 (71%) children were premature, 27 (26.2) children were premature and 3 (2.9%) children were preterm (Table 3.1.2.).

Table 3.1.2.

Оценка анамнестических данных детей в исследовании

Анамнестический критерий	Основная группа n=103	Контрольная группа n=20
Удовлетворительное состояние при рождении	44	16
Среднетяжелое состояние при рождении	51	-
Тяжелое состояние при рождении	5	-
Реанимационные мероприятия с последующей ИВЛ от 2 до 7 суток	2	-
Доношенность	73	18
Недоношенность I степени (34–37 недель гестации)	27	2
Переношенность (более 42 недель)	3	-

The role of indicators assessed by the Apgar scale in the first 5 minutes was analysed in the development of ARP. In this case, in 49 children of the main group, the Apgar scale was 7-8 points, in 47 children 5-6 points (mild asphyxia), and in 4 children 3-4 points (medium level of asphyxia), which reflected to what extent the infants' brain hypoxia was in the first minutes. (Figure 3.1.1.).

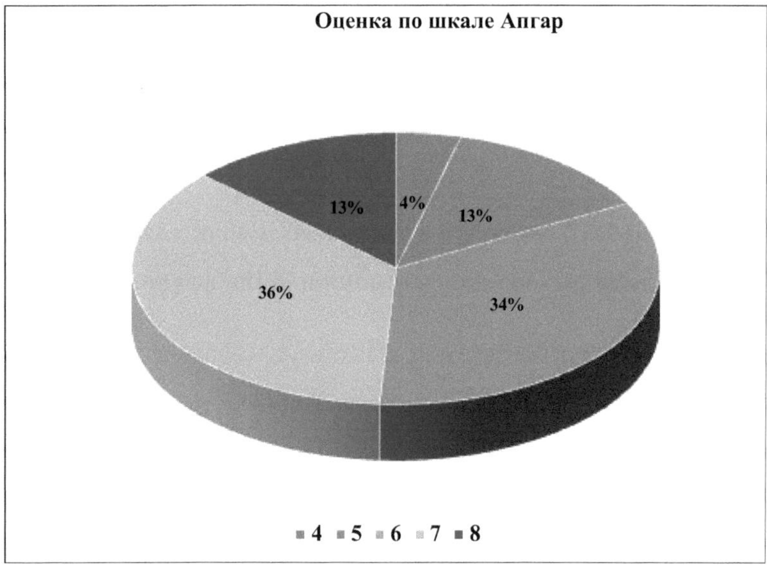

Fig.3.1.1 Comparative characterisation of risk factors in the perinatal period (condition of the child at birth)

When studying the neonatal period (Fig. 3.1.2.) (child's condition during the neonatal period), 85% of children had perinatal CNS damage of hypoxic genesis (in the form of cerebral excitability syndrome, cerebral depression syndrome, motor dystonia syndrome, Vascular vascular distention syndrome), 25% had intrauterine dystrophy (hypotrophy), 28% had perinatal (intrauterine) infection, and 8% had jaundice before 1 month of age.

Патология неонатального периода
перинатальное поражение ЦНС
82,5%
внутриутробная дистрофия (гипотрофия)
27,2%
перинатальная (внутриутробная) инфекция
27,2%
желтухи до 1 месяца
7,8%
0,0%
20,0%
40,0%
60,0%
80,0%
100,0%

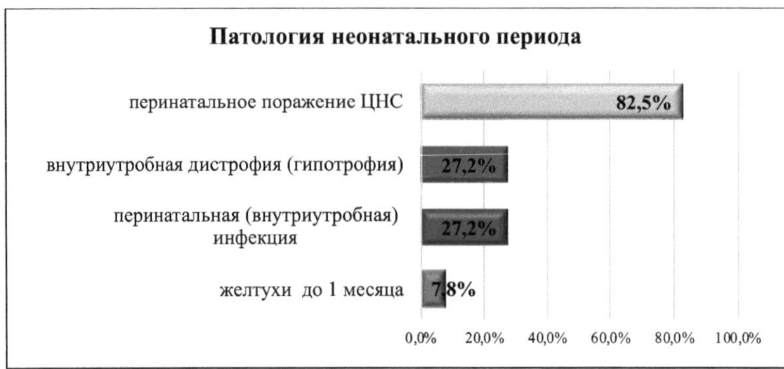

Fig.3.1.2 Comparative characterisation of risk factors in the perinatal period (child's condition in the newborn period)

As a result of our research, concomitant somatic pathology was registered in 90.2% of ARP children. Pathology of the respiratory system, pathology of the cardiovascular system and gastrointestinal tract were the most frequently observed.

Diseases of respiratory and ENT organs were detected in 48.5% of patients, among which the most frequently registered were out-of-hospital bronchopneumonia (37.6% of patients) and acute rhinosinusitis (11.9% of patients).

Among the diseases of the gastrointestinal tract organs, acute and chronic gastroduodenitis (35.6%), biliary dyskinesia (15.4%) and dysbacteriosis (56.7%) were most frequently detected in patients with ARP.

Analysis of the results of the study showed that of 23.8% of patients with confirmed pathology of the cardiovascular system, sinus node dysfunction was the most frequent - sinus tachy- and bradyarrhythmias in 11.5% of patients, transient atrioventricular (AV) block of the first degree and (AV) block of the second degree were detected equally often in 12.4% of cases in children of the main groups.

The combination of several pathologies was more frequent in the main group of children and accounted for 66.8%, while in the control group combined pathology was significantly less frequent and accounted for 5% ($p < 0.05$). The results of objective examination are systematised in Table 3.1.3.

Table 3.1.3.

Results of the comparative analysis of the main group on the aggravation of somatic anamnesis

Indicator	ARP Cyanotic form n=47	ARP Pale mould n=22	ARP Mixed form N=34
Skin diseases	3	1	2
Diseases of the gastrointestinal tract (GI tract)	13	16	14
Functional bowel disorders	10	20	18
Respiratory and ENT diseases	35	19	32
Chronic and subacute infection	12	7	11
Iron deficiency anaemia (IDA)	38	22	30
Rakhitis	36	20	34
Diseases of the cardiovascular system	1	2	4
Diseases of the visual organs	2	1	8

When analysing the data presented in Table 3.1.3, somatic diseases were diagnosed in all forms of ARP. However, in the cyanotic form, diseases of ENT organs, iron deficiency anaemia and rickets were more frequent.

When studying the family history, we obtained information taking into account the hereditary condition of ARP, where we found that 23% of children in the main group had a paternally aggravated heredity. 77% of hereditary history was not aggravated. The comparison data on ARP heredity are presented in Fig. 3.1.3.

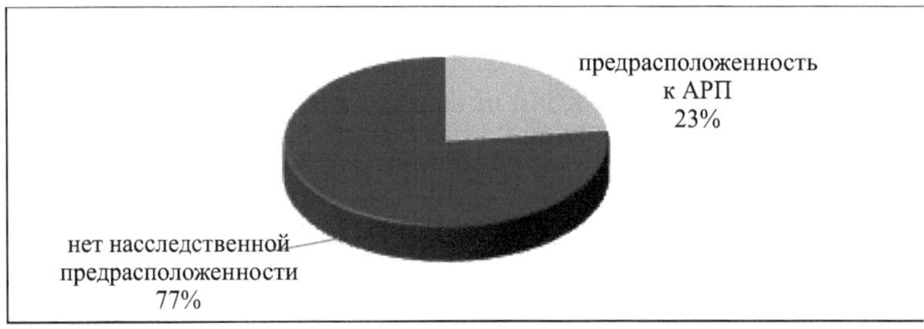

Fig.3.1.3 Comparative characterisation of ARP depending on the presence of hereditary predisposition to ARP

§3.2 Results of the clinical examination of ARPs

ARPs have their specific features and therefore we studied in detail the debut, nature, course, frequency of paroxysms and factors provoking these attacks.

When we examined the history data, the frequency of affective-respiratory paroxysms in 52.4% of children started at the age of 3-12 months, 29.1% of children at the age of 13-24 months and 18.4% of children were noted to have seizures at the age of 25-36 months (Figure 3.2.1).

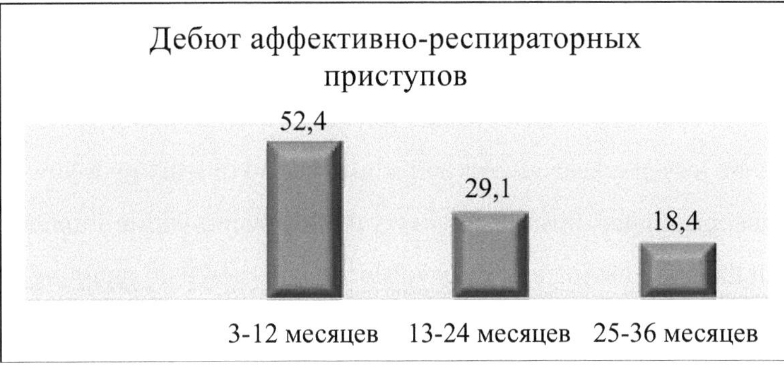

Fig.3.2.1 Comparative characteristics of ARP depending on the time of the first manifestation of seizures

In the research work, we divided the children of the main group into the following forms depending on the nature of the paroxysm. The diagnosis is based on a characteristic and stereotypical sequence of clinical events that begin with provocation leading to crying or emotional distress, silent state of exhalation accompanied by colour change. As shown in the table, cyanotic form of ARP was more diagnosed in 45.6% of children, pale form in 21.3% of children and mixed form in 33.0% of children (Table 3.2.1.).

Tables 3.2.1.

Distribution of seizures by type in children with affective-respiratory paroxysm

Seizures by type	n=103 (%)
Cyanotic	45,6
Pale	21,3
Mixed	33,0

Cyanotic BPH attacks were often provoked by emotional stimuli such as anger - 39 (84.7%) children and 8 (17.3%) frustration. The child usually cries vigorously but usually for less than 15 seconds, then holds his breath on exhalation. Apnoea is associated with rapid onset of cyanosis. Some episodes may resolve at this point, but there may be loss of consciousness and a brief period of lethargy followed by an opisthotonic posture. Recovery usually occurs within 1 minute, with the child having a few convulsive breaths and then returning to normal breathing and consciousness.

Pale ARP attacks were usually provoked by sudden fright - 12 (54.5%) and pain - 8 (36.7%). Sometimes the provoking factor was a fall with mild head trauma. Sometimes, the provoking event was not observed and the child was found already in the episode. The child gasps and cries, usually this does not last long. The child then becomes quiet, loses consciousness and becomes pale with perspiration. Clonic limb movements and urinary incontinence may occur in more severe episodes. Cyanosis may occur during an attack, but it is much milder than in cyanotic attacks of breath-holding. The child usually regains consciousness in less than 1 minute but may sleep for several hours after the episode.

Depending on the severity of the course of ARP attacks, patients were divided into 3 subgroups (mild-33%, moderate-29.1%, severe-19.4%) (Table 3.2.2.).

Table 3.2.2.

Distribution of examined children depending on the severity of the course of APR attacks.

ARP		
light	medium	heavy
39 (37,8%)	35 (33,9%)	29 (28,1%)

The attacks in ARP patients proceeded as follows: attacks of freezing on the background of crying, accompanied by cyanosis of the face (20 cases) or pallor (6 cases), followed by short-term loss of consciousness and sometimes mild tremor of the limbs (6 cases); the attacks manifested as a brief tilt of the head backwards with crying or dystonic postures, impaired coordination and periodic vomiting (10 cases); attacks of tonic tension of muscles of the lower limbs, facing inwards or crossed, with sweating, sometimes staring and brief freezing (18 cases); attacks of freezing against the background of crying, cyanosis of the face (27 cases) or pallor accompanied by tonic tension of the trunk (16 cases) and/or limbs, without loss of consciousness (Fig.3.2.2.).

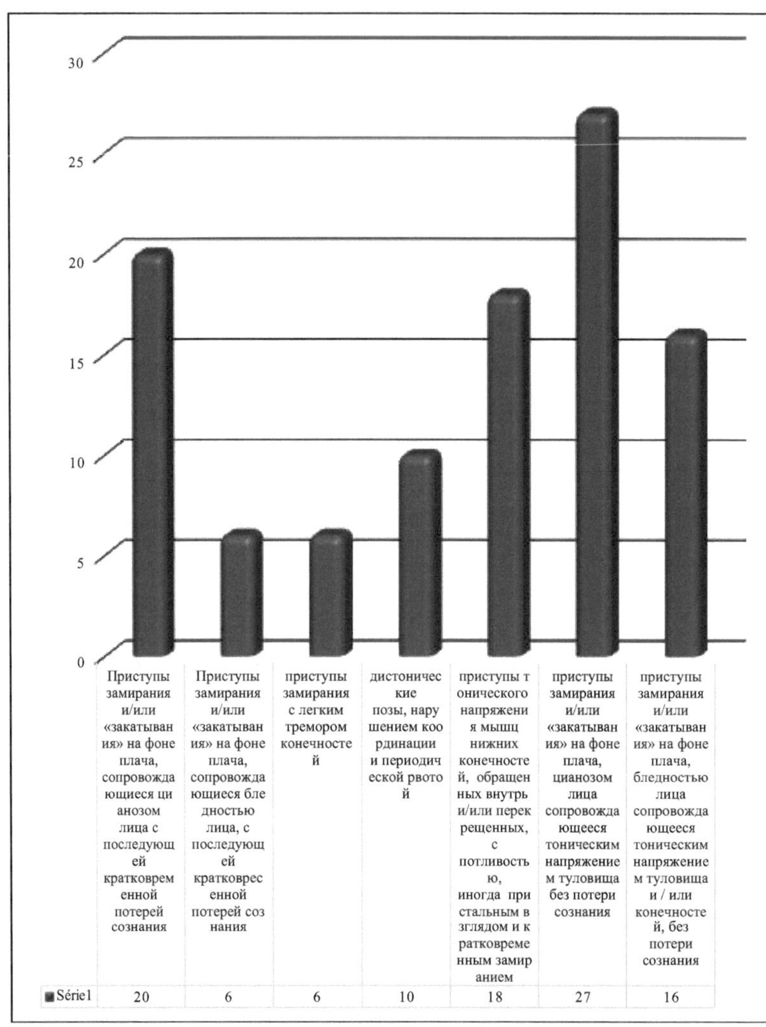

Fig.3.2.2 Comparative characteristics of ARP depending on the clinical course of seizures

A detailed history and examination are important in making the diagnosis and in differentiating them from epileptic seizures and other causes of syncope.

Depending on the disturbance of consciousness during ARP attacks, patients were divided into - with and without disturbance of consciousness (Table 3.2.3.).

Table 3.2.3.

Clinical characteristics of paroxysmal states, depending on the presence of disturbance of consciousness

	Cyanotic n=47 (45,6%)			**Pale n=22 (21,3%)**			**Mixed n=34 (33,0%)**		
	light	medium	heavy	light	medium	heavy	light	medium	heavy
From the offence. consciousn esses	-	10	10	1	2	3	-	2	2
No violation consciousn esses	12	10	5	5	6	5	1 7	8	5

The number of seizures in children with affective-respiratory paroxysm depending on the recurrence of seizures was selected weekly. 20.4% of children had 3 attacks per week, 26.2% of children had 5 attacks per week, and the remaining 53.4% of children had 1 attack per week (Fig.3.2.3.).

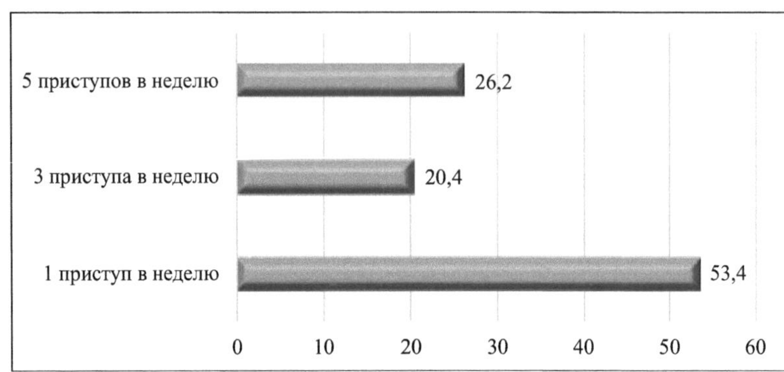

Fig.3.2.3 Comparative characteristic of ARP depending on on the frequency of seizures per week

When studying the clinical and neurological characteristics of patients with ARP, syndromes characteristic of central nervous system lesions in the perinatal period were identified. The syndrome of increased neuro-reflex excitability in the cyanotic form of ARP was detected in 12 children, and in the mixed form of ARP the syndrome of emotional and behavioural disorders was detected with equal frequency (Tab.3.2.4. Fig.3.2.4.).

Table 3.2.4.

Characteristics of neurological syndromes in the examined children by ARP types

Indicator	Cyanotic	Pale	Mixed
No special features	2 (1,9%)	4 (3,9%)	2 (1,9%)
The syndrome of increased neuro-reflex excitability	12 (11,6%)	5 (4,9%)	6 95,8%)
Hypertension-hydrocephalus syndrome.	4 (3,9%)	1 (0,9%)	1 (0,9%)

Cerebral depression syndrome	6 (5,8%)	2 (1,9%)	2 (1,9%)
Autonomic-visceral dysfunction syndrome	8 (7,8%)	3 (2,9%)	4 (3,9%)
Delayed stages of psychomotor development	9 (8,7%)	2 (1,9%)	7 (6,8%)
Emotional and behavioural disorders	6 (5,8%)	5 (4,9%)	12 (11,7%)

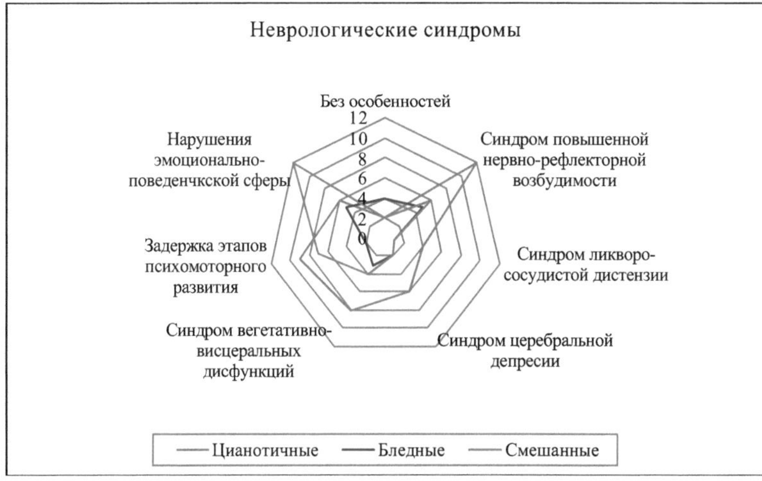

Fig.3.2.4 Comparative characteristics of neurological syndromes in children by ARP types

Clinical and neurological examination of children in the main group revealed the following neurological symptoms: divergent strabismus in 3 (2.9%) children, convergence disorders in 4 (3.9%) children, nasolabial fold smoothing in 7 (6.8%) children, mild tongue deviation in 3 (2.9%) children, muscular hypotonia in 27 (26,2%) children, muscle dystonia in 23 (22.3%) children, muscle hypertonia in 16 (15.5%) children, strengthening of deep tendon reflexes in 36

(34.5%) children, suppression of deep tendon reflexes in 14 (13.6%) children. It was revealed that the frequency of sleep disorders (dyssomnia, insomnia, somnolongia, somnambulism, nightmares) was significantly ($p<0.05$) higher in children with ARP - 65 (63.1%) (Fig.3.2.5).

расстройства сна
65
угнетение глубоких сухожильных...
14
усиление глубоких сухожильных...
36
мышечная гипертония
16
мышечная дистония
23
мышечная гипотония
27
легкая девиация языка
3
сглаженность носогубных складок
7
нарушения конвергенции
4
косоглазие
3

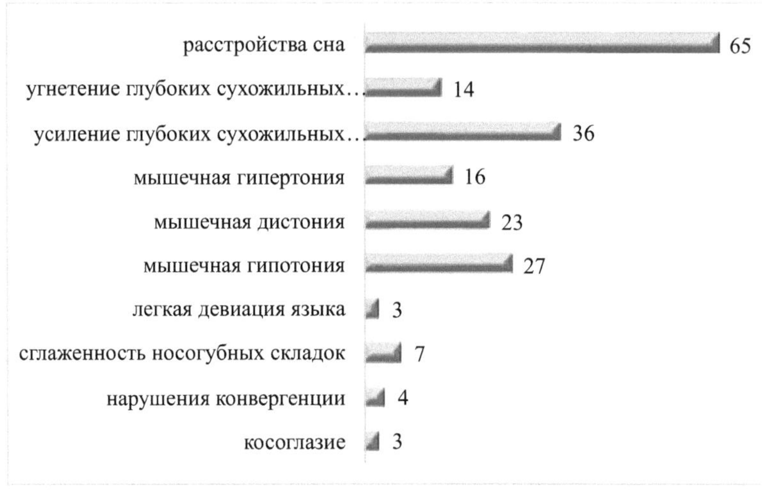

Fig.3.2.5. Comparative characteristics of neurological symptoms in children by ARP types

Neuropsychological assessment is an indispensable tool because it is a method that includes several systematised procedures to study and map mental and cognitive functions related to the functioning of the central nervous system. It analyses the presence of behavioural changes due to neurological dysfunction or cognitive difficulties caused by developmental disorders and brain lesions. The neuropsychological assessment consists of a detailed study that performs the function of assessing cognitive, language, perceptual and psychomotor indicators in order to correlate these indicators with functional and structural brain states. For this purpose the methodology of Pantyukhin G.V., Pechora K.L., Frucht E.L. (2007) was used.

Motor skill development involves important interactions between the child and his or her environment. It also involves complex interactions between the physical and genetic systems (especially reflexes) present at birth, the child's sensory, emotional, social and cognitive development, which is largely learnt or constructed. Psychomotor development is related to general motor skills (e.g., learning to walk) and fine motor skills (e.g., holding a spoon). When motor development was tested (fine motor skills) in (36.8%) of children, (large motor skills) in (26.2%) of children in the main group, there was a delay of 1 epicrisis period. This motor development is continuously linked to sensory development, with which it functions in constant interaction. For example, to grasp an object, the child must coordinate his gaze and grip. In the study of sensory development (visual and auditory orienting reactions) in (11.6%) children of the main group there was a delay of 1 epicrisis term. When testing the function of active speech in (33.9%) children and understanding of addressed speech in (15.5%) children of the main group there was a delay of 1 epicrisis term.

Neuropsychological study showed that the indicators of social skills acquisition in children: development of play ability in children (25.2%), constructive activity in children (11.6%) and pictorial activity in children (26.2%) lagged behind by 1 epicrisis period compared to children in the comparison group ($p>0.05$), these changes are associated with poor development of fine motor skills.

Children with ARD who scored significantly low on the Emotional Sphere measure took a long time to come out of any negative emotional state, even when they were comforted by their mothers. This, of course, forced their parents to take drastic measures to please them. The groups of control children could be easily distracted from their bad moods and they responded better to their mother's calls during play compared to the ARP children ($p>0.05$). So, we hypothesise that children with ARP have a 'tendency to stay' in their peak emotional states. Our study clearly showed that children with affective-respiratory paroxysms differ from other children in that they are more sensitive, reacting sharply and intensely to any negative environment.

Thus, the neuropsychodiagnostic study in children with affective-respiratory paroxysms revealed a lag in sensory and speech development and impaired fine motor skills (Fig. 3.2.6.).

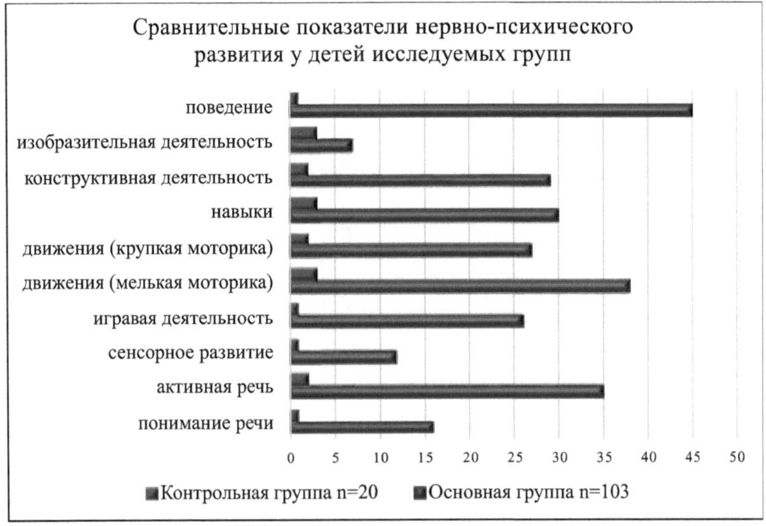

Fig.3.2.6. Comparative indicators of psychomotor development in children of the studied groups.

Neurophysiology continues to study the pathogenesis of affective-respiratory attacks, but emphasises their unconditional connection with age-related features of the central nervous system and, to a greater extent, with ANS function. Studying the peculiarities of the autonomic state in ARP will help further treatment. Sympathetic and parasympathetic nervous circuits coordinate stress responses and anti-stress responses, respectively. Balance between these systems leads to homeostasis, whereas imbalance leads to pathological states. Therefore, we evaluated the initial vegetative tone in children using A.M. Vein's table. A change in any type of vegetative tone can affect the development of clinical signs of ARP. The results of the initial vegetative tone assessment were eutonia in 27 children, sympathicotonia in 45 children and vagotonia in 15 children (Fig.3.2.7.).

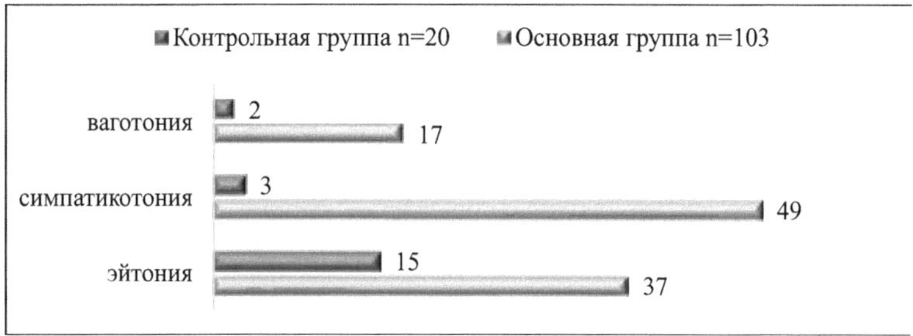

Fig.3.2.7. Comparative indices of initial vegetative tone in children of the studied groups.

When assessing the vegetative reactivity of the children of the main group using the telt-test, it was found that 35 (33.9%) children had hypersympathicotonic vegetative reactivity, 15 (14.5%) children had asympathicotonic vegetative reactivity and 50 (48.5%) children had normotonic vegetative reactivity; normotonic vegetative reactivity was found in all children of the control group (Fig.3.2.8.).

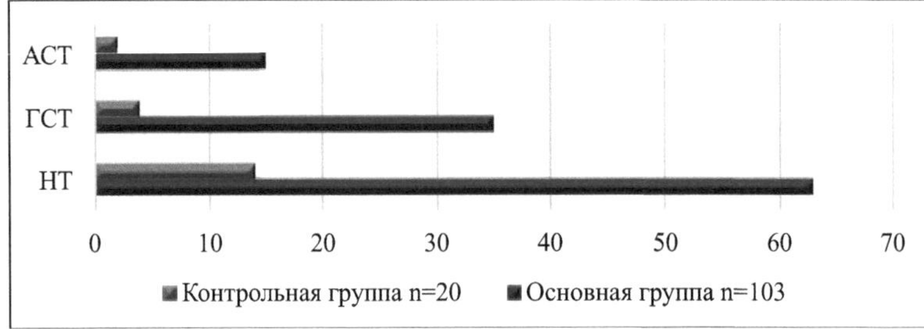

Fig.3.2.8. Comparative indices of vegetative reactivity in children of the studied groups.

§3.3 Neurosonographic findings

To detect age-appropriate structural lesions of the brain, children underwent a screening NSG examination.

In 58.9% of children with ARP, various brain lesions were detected by NSG. The most frequently detected changes on NSG data were: dilation of the external or internal liquor spaces (36.8%), asymmetry of the lateral ventricles (18.4%), widening of the interhemispheric gap (17.4%), subatrophic changes of the brain substance (15.5%), and lenticulostriary vasculopathy (1.9%).

Neuroimaging data (neurosonography) are shown in **Table 3.3.1.**

Morphological changes in the brain	**Main group n (%)**	**Control group n (%)**
Norma	29,1	85
Enlargement of external or internal liquor spaces	36,8	5

Asymmetry of the lateral ventricles	18,4	
Expansion of interhemispheric gaps	17,4	10
Subatrophic changes brain matter	15,5	
Lenticulostriary vasculopathy	1,9%	

In children with ARP, the characteristic features of brain lesions are posthypoxic changes in the form of disruption of the liquor pathways. In most cases, hypoxic-ischaemic lesions of the CNS detected in children correspond to the 2nd degree with the predominance of neuro-reflex excitability syndrome in the clinic, and unfavourable pregnancy and childbirth play a major role in their development.

§3.4 Electroencephalography findings in children with ARP

EEG analysis is based on pathophysiological interpretation of the data and diagnostic conclusion about damage to certain brain structures and the nature of the pathological process. When recording EEG, the characteristics of biopotentials were taken into account, namely their nature, frequency, amplitude, localisation, dominant rhythm, interhemispheric asymmetry, frequency of zonal differences, degree of synchronisation of biorhythms along different pathways and paroxysmal pathological processes. The frequency of α-rhythm was significantly lower in the majority of children with ARP. Bioelectrical activity in the α-rhythm range was represented by bursts lasting up to several seconds, while the intervals between α-rhythm bursts were filled with flat EEG, with generalised bursts of slow-wave activity observed against a background of normal electrical activity, mainly in the central leads.

On EEG, the hypersynchronous slowing of background activity was accompanied by a diffuse background electrical reduction for 15 s and high-amplitude symmetrical rhythmic discharges in the anterior regions of the head for about 8 s.

No specific EEG phenomena were detected. However, asymmetry of α-rhythm, is not always pathological. Thus, in our study, asymmetry was recorded in children with ARP in 32% (n=33).

In children of the control group in the majority of cases, β-rhythms were registered in the area of the anterior central gyrus, in children with ARP localisation of β-rhythms in the posterior central and frontal gyrus was 20.4% (n=21).

Generalised bilateral-synchronous bursts of high-amplitude θ-, δ-waves, predominantly expressed in the central parietal in 12 (11.6%) children, parieto-occipital in 21 (20.4%) children were detected. In terms of the frequency of θ- and δ-rhythms, we obtained the following results: in the control groups these indices were 4.73±0.16 and 1.73±0.14, and in children with ARP - 6.15±0.1 and 2.2±0.12, respectively.

In our study, we evaluated EEG indices depending on the severity of paroxysms. To determine the relationship between the severity of paroxysms and the indices of bioelectrical activity of the brain. Thus, 14.5% of children with mild forms of ARP had age norm, 13.7% of children had signs of dysfunction of nonspecific median brain structures, and the remaining 5.8% of children showed diffuse changes in brain bioelectrical activity in the form of disorganisation of α-rhythm. The data obtained are summarised in *diagram -3.4.1*

возрастная норма
14,5
дезорганизации а-ритма
5,8
признаки дисфункции неспецифических срединных структур головного мозга.
13,7

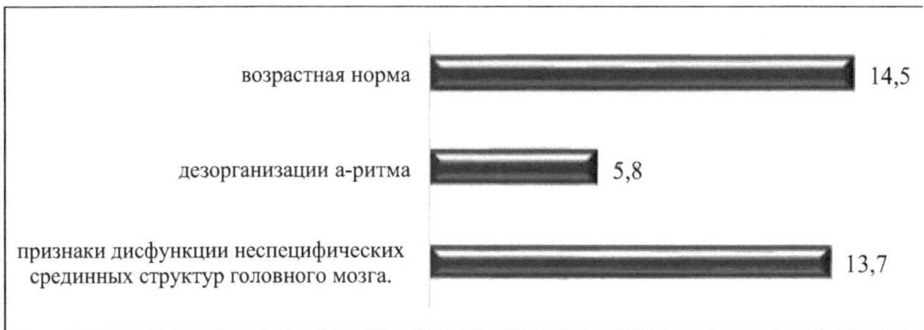

Fig.3.4.1 Comparative indices of brain bioelectrical activity in mild forms of ARP.

In 34.5% of children with severe ARP, there was a generalised high-amplitude slowing of EEG activity at 4-5 Hz (θ-band), followed by an increase in brainwave amplitude with a decrease in frequency at 1.5-3 Hz (δ-band). Return to the supine position was associated with a decrease in brainwave amplitude and an increase in frequency to 4-5 Hz, followed by restoration of normal EEG and arousal patterns (mean total syncope duration 23.2 seconds) (Figure-3.4.2.).

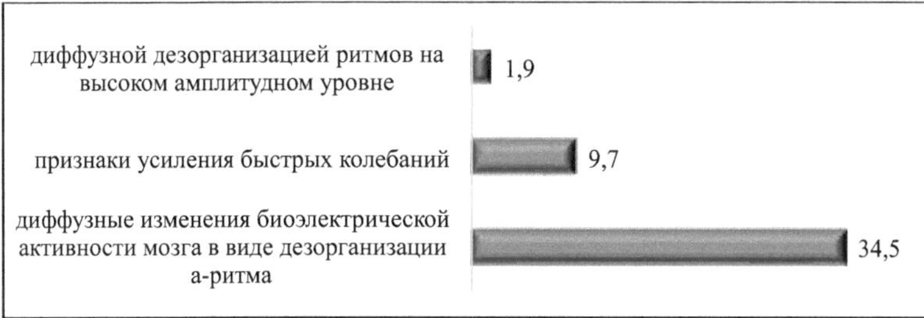

Fig.3.4.2 Comparative indices of brain bioelectrical activity in severe forms of ARP.

In 14.1% of patients with moderately severe forms of ARP, there was a generalised slowing of high-amplitude EEG in the θ-band, followed by an increase in brainwave amplitude and slowing in the δ-band. This was followed by a sudden decrease in brainwave amplitude, resulting in the disappearance of brain activity ("flat" EEG). Returning to the supine position neither immediately resolved the EEG abnormalities nor restored consciousness, both of which occurred after an additional time interval (mean total syncope duration 41.4 seconds) (Figure-3.4.3.).

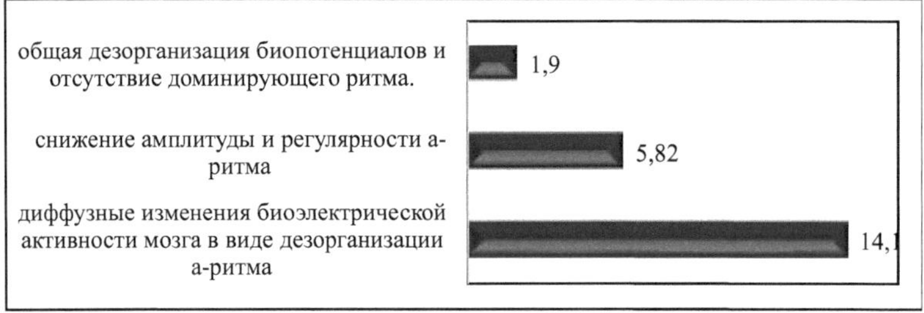

Fig.3.4.3 Comparative indices of brain bioelectrical activity in moderate forms of ARP.

Returning to the supine position did not result in immediate elimination of EEG abnormalities, but complete normalisation of brain activity occurred after an additional time interval (mean duration 15.1±6.0 seconds; range 7 to 22 seconds). The prevalence of tonic-clonic twitches during loss of consciousness was significantly higher in patients with pale forms of ARP (20 of 22; 90.9%) compared with patients with cyanotic forms of ARP (14 of 46; 30.4%, $P<0.01$). In all cases, no spike or spike-wave activity, lateralising or focal abnormalities could be detected in any child.

At the end of the test, the EEG was found to be normal in all cases, and no epileptic abnormality was noted in any patient despite the occurrence of syncopal episodes.

Conclusions to Chapter III:

A high frequency of perinatal risk factors for nervous system damage in ARP has been established.

The results of the study showed that among the examined patients the most frequent somatic pathologies were diseases of the respiratory system and ENT organs, digestive organs, as well as pathology of the cardiovascular system.

The appearance of neurological symptoms in children with ARP is associated with central nervous system damage in the perinatal period. A polymorphism of symptoms and syndromes accompanied by changes in tendon reflexes, muscle tone and hMN lesions was observed depending on the severity of the perinatal period.

When studying the activity of the autonomic nervous system in children of the main group with ARP, an increase in sympathetic tone was found.

The neurobehavioural study showed that children in the main group with ARP lagged behind in sensory and motor development.

In children, ARP on EEG was predominant in all areas of α-rhythm, β-activity of low frequency in all age groups. The main disturbances of bioelectrical activity in the range of alpha rhythm, generalised flashes of slow-wave activity, mainly in the central leads, against the background of normal electrical activity remained. On the

EEG, hypersynchronous slowing of background activity was accompanied by diffuse background electrical reduction for 15 s and high-amplitude symmetrical rhythmic discharges in the anterior regions of the head for about 8 s.

CHAPTER IV. VALUES OF BIOCHEMICAL BIOMARKERS OF OXIDATIVE STRESS IN CHILDREN WITH ARP

§4.1 Biochemical results

The peroxidant-antioxidant system of blood serum was assessed by the level of malonic dialdehyde (MDA), diene conjugates (DC), superoxide dismutase (SOD), glutathione peroxidase, glutathione reductase, catalase, cytochrome-C and nitric oxide (NO) activity determined by spectrophotometric method (L.P. Andreeva et al, 1988; Dubinin B.B. et al., 1983)

The results of the study of POL processes in blood plasma in ARP children revealed that MDA and DC indices at mild course of attacks show 3.09±0.4, 1.77±0.21 to the levels of control values 2.97±0.11, 1.65±0.04 ($p<0.01$), in patients with moderate and severe clinical course these indices are significantly higher ($p<0.001$) than in control children (Table 4.4.1.).

Table 4.1.1.

Comparative indices of plasma POL in patients with ARP

Analysed groups of children	POL indicators analysed	
	MDA mmol/ml	DK
Mild ARP n= 34	3.09±0.4*	1.77±0.21**
Moderately severe ARP n= 30	3.14±0.05*	1.81±0.01*
Severe ARP n=20	4.68±0.23***	1.95±0.08***
Healthy n=20	2.97±0.11*	1.65±0.04

*P<0.01; **P<0.03; ***P<0.001; - reliability of differences with control parameters.

As can be seen from Table 4.4.1, the accumulation of POL products in blood plasma and erythrocytes increased with increasing severity of ARP attacks or, on the contrary, the increase of POL products in blood aggravated the attacks.

Oxidative breakdown of biological phospholipids occurs in most cell membranes, including mitochondria, microsomes, peroxisomes and the plasma membrane. The toxicity of lipid peroxidation products is usually associated with neurotoxicity; enhancement of this process exacerbates seizures.

In the metabolism of every cell, an oxidation reaction takes place. The presence of oxygen in the internal environment is, on the one hand, important for cell function; on the other hand, it is a threat that causes oxidative damage due to the formation of free radicals Superoxide dismutase is the only antioxidant enzyme that removes the superoxide anion, converting this free radical to oxygen and hydrogen peroxide, thus preventing the formation of peroxynitrite and further damage.

The study of antioxidant defence parameters revealed their decrease. The content of AOS parameters in blood plasma of children in the main group decreased with increasing severity of ARP attacks ($p<0.01$).

Our findings suggest that decreased SOD activity and levels in children with affective-respiratory paroxysms make them more susceptible to oxidative damage caused by reactive oxygen species (ROS) (Table 4.1.2).

Table 4.1.2.

Comparative indices of AOS in patients with ARP

Analysed groups of children	AOS indicators analysed				
	Catalase µ	Superoxid e	Glutathio ne	Glutathio ne	Glutathi one

	Cat/mg protein	dismutase units/mg protein	reductase mM/min gr protein	peroxidase mM/min gr protein	transferase mM/min gr protein
Mild ARP n= 34	39.11±0.09	10.03±0.1	1.63±0.5	1.90±0.2	3.33±0.1 **
Moderately severe ARP n= 30	38.98±1.01	9.9±0.4	1.59±1.03	1.88±0.6	2.78±0.8 *
Severe ARP n=20	36.48±1.72*	9.53±0.42***	1.35±0.04	1.84±0.02	2.33±0.11
Healthy n=20	43.42±2.77	12.32±0.27	1.78±0.02	2.06±0.05	3,75±0.18

*P<0.05; **P<0.01; ***P<0.001- reliability of differences with control values.

The above data show that patients with ARP had decreased content of AOS enzymes in blood, increased amount of POL products, indicating cell membrane damage.

These facts may be due to the fact that oxidative stress products can cause damage to brain cells, which can lead to the development of paroxysms.

Cytochrome-C-oxidase, a member of the haemo-Cu oxidases, is the end enzyme of the mitochondrial electron transport chain, essential for the transfer of electrons to the terminal electron acceptor, oxygen. In addition to its role in electron transport in conjunction with proton gradient formation, it is thought to have an important function in regulating the entire system. Cytochrome-C-oxidase is a useful endogenous metabolic marker for neurons as the nervous system is highly dependent on aerobic metabolism for energy supply, plays an essential role in mitochondrial aerobic energy metabolism. During the study, it was observed that serum cytochrome-C-oxidase level was found to be diagnostically significant in predicting affective-respiratory paroxysm. The amount of cytochrome-C-oxidase was significantly reduced in severe ARP compared to its mild form ($p<0.01$) (Table 4.1.3.). Based on this, we can predict that decreased cytochrome-C-oxidase levels exacerbate seizures may also lead to epileptic seizure.

Table 4.1.3.

Comparative indices of cytochrome C-oxidase enzyme activity in the blood of healthy children and patients with ARP in comparative aspect (µmol/mg protein)

№	Analysed groups of children	n	µmol/mg protein
1	Lightweight ARP	34	1.65±0.2
2	Moderately severe ARP	30	1.45±0.12
3	Severe ARP	20	1.33±0.04**
4	Healthy	20	1.78±0.02

**P<0.01- reliability of differences with control parameters.

We studied the content of nitric oxide metabolites in blood plasma to identify risk factors for the development of ARP. A significant increase in the content of NO metabolites was observed in children of the main groups ($p=0.025$), which also indicated the presence of marked cerebral hypoxia. Given its unique characteristics of vasodilation (improving blood flow and oxygen supply) and modulation of energy metabolism, nitric oxide (NO) is the main signalling and effector molecule mediating the body's response to hypoxia. We have identified a key role for NO in the adaptation of the organism to an acute mismatch in energy demand (Table 4.1.4.).

Table 4.1.4.

Nitric oxide *NOx* metabolites in the plasma of healthy children and patients (µmol/l)

№	Analysed groups of children	n	*NOx* content, µmol/L	min	max	median
1	Lightweight ARP	34	42.5 ± 1.02	19.01	65.71	30.2
2	Moderately severe ARP	30	54.63 ± 0.80	21.15	75.7	42.54
3	Severe ARP	20	68.06 ± 8.16*	25.32	190.39	57.64
4	Healthy	20	34.95 ± 2.30	18.08	66.87	31.19

*P<0.05 - reliability of differences with control indices.

Micronutrient deficiency to some extent provokes the development of ARP. For this purpose, a general blood analysis of patients was performed to detect iron deficiency anaemia. Total erythrocyte haemoglobin averaged 80.5±4.2 in children of the main group and in the control group this index was 108.6±3.52, mean erythrocyte count was 3.02±0.1 and 3.85±0.09, mean colour index was 0.78±0.01 and 0.98±0.04. The listed indices are statistically reliable ($p<0.01$).

As a result of blood analysis, iron deficiency anaemia of the II degree was detected in 18 children with severe ARP, in 12 children with moderately severe ARP, and in 5 children with mild ARP. Grade I iron deficiency anaemia was detected in 68 children (Fig.4.1.1.).

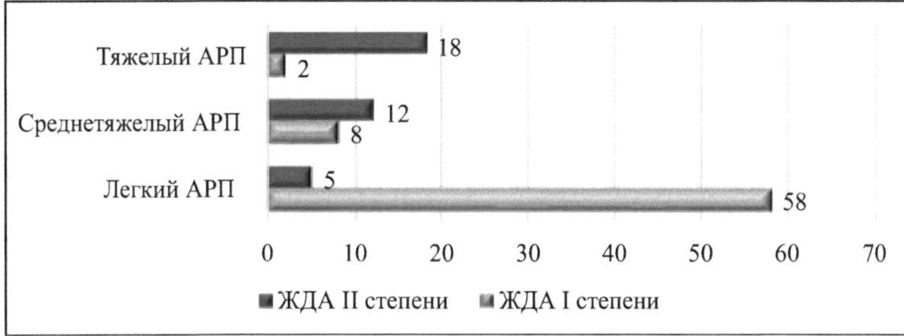

Figure 4.1.1 Distribution of children according to haematological parameters

The results of biochemical study showed that the oxidant-antioxidant balance in children with ARP was disturbed in favour of oxidants, depending on the form and frequency of attacks per day. The more severe the seizure was, the lower the blood AOS was found to be. In addition, the presence of WDD was found to be associated with increased oxidative stress in children with ARP, especially at the erythrocyte level; among the oxidant parameters erythrocyte MDA and DC, erythrocyte SOD and antioxidant parameters, they are the biomarkers that show the highest probability of having an ARP attack and increased frequency of apnoea attacks. We found that children with ARP had significantly higher malonic dialdehyde ($p<0.001$) and lower serum glutathione peroxide ($p<0.001$) and superoxide dismutase ($p<0.001$) levels than children in the control group. The data suggest that dysregulation of oxidative and antioxidant systems may play a role in the pathophysiology of ARP.

Our studies have shown that changes in AOS and POL parameters in blood in young children with ARP form the pathophysiological basis for the development of non-epileptic paroxysms, can be an additional diagnostic criterion and have prognostic value for epileptic seizures.

Conclusions to Chapter IV:

The results of the biochemical study showed that the oxidant-antioxidant balance in children with ARP is disturbed in favour of oxidants, depending on the form and frequency of attacks per day.

In cerebral hypoxia, active metabolic processes begin, leading to an increase in free radical oxidation. Free radicals penetrate cells and try to snatch an electron from another, defenceless molecule. When molecules in the body's tissues are forced to give up their electrons to free radicals, their cells are damaged. As a result of this action, free radicals can initiate a chain reaction: because if a new reactant is also released as a free radical, it can cause a similar reaction. Cells damaged in this way either die or change in a dangerous way.

Thus, these chain reactions can result in damage to DNA and RNA within the cell, the cell membrane, and many other important molecules in the cellular environment. This, in turn, can contribute to the development of diseases.

As mentioned earlier, active radicals can cause oxidative damage to lipids in the body. This damage primarily affects lipid membranes, especially the unsaturated fatty acids in them. The resulting chain reaction results in the accumulation of lipid peroxides in the cell membrane. Ultimately, this leads to loss of structural integrity and, consequently, to disruption of normal cellular functions.

But not only lipids of cell membranes, but also lipoproteins in plasma can undergo oxidative damage. The data suggest that dysregulation of oxidative and antioxidant systems may play a role in the pathophysiology of ARP.

CHAPTER V. PECULIARITIES OF TACTICS OF MANAGEMENT OF CHILDREN WITH ARP

The next stage was to determine the effectiveness of the therapy. In our study, in addition to basic antioxidant therapy, iron preparations and melatonin, which has membrane- and cytoprotective and antioxidant effects, were used. Melatonin may serve as a potential therapeutic free radical scavenger and broad-spectrum antioxidant (activation of antioxidant pathways). Its antioxidant effects are thought to be much stronger than those of vitamins E and C and glutathione. The molecule can capture up to 10 AFCs (reactive oxygen species) compared to classical antioxidants, which neutralise one or fewer AFCs. The protective effect of melatonin is to increase the activity of antioxidant enzymes including superoxide dismutase (SOD), catalase (K) and glutathione peroxidase (GPO) by increasing the expression of the aforementioned enzymes [75;1-9-c]. In addition, melatonin is located on the surface of cell membranes near the polar heads of phospholipids, consequently protecting cell membranes from oxidation. By altering the fluidity of membranes, it removes radicals before they damage the lipids and proteins of the cell membrane. Melatonin does not have pro-oxidant properties. Sleep problems in children with affective-respiratory paroxysms may be related to abnormal circadian melatonin secretion, insufficient melatonin production, or melatonin receptor insensitivity. Sleep disorders are the most common problems in the paediatric population. Sleep deprivation at the cellular level increases oxidative stress in the hippocampus and leads to loss of synaptic connections of neurons, which can affect neurocognitive disorders, especially attention, behavioural and emotional aspects of development.

Children with affective-respiratory paroxysms received melatonin (Melglis) in age-appropriate doses. The list of treatment efficacy indicators is given in Table 5.1. Registration of the study data efficacy indicators was performed immediately after treatment. Treatment efficacy was evaluated one month after the start of therapy.

Table 5.1.

List of indicators of the effectiveness of treatment of children with paroxysms

0 point	Lack of efficiency	No reduction in the frequency and duration of ARF attacks was observed after treatment.
1 point	Low efficiency	Slight reduction in the frequency and duration of BPH attacks after treatment.
2 points	Average efficiency	Significant reduction in the frequency and duration of BPH attacks after treatment.
3 points	High efficiency	A dramatic reduction in the frequency and duration of BPH attacks after treatment.

Examining the status of children with ARP after pathogenetic treatment using quantitative scores will help determine the effectiveness of treatment (Table 5.2).

Table 5.2.

Comparative assessment of the effectiveness of treatment methods

	Scheme A (n=60)	Scheme B (34)
Lack of efficiency	3	3

Low efficiency	17	12
Average efficiency	27	16
High efficiency	13	3
Total score	2,9±0,08*	2,1±0,11

*p<0.05 - reliability between the compared groups

As can be seen from this table, medium and high efficacy of melatonin (Melglis) was observed in 40 (66.7%) children, low efficacy in 17 (28.3%) children, and insufficient efficacy was observed in 3 (5%) children.

The effect of melatonin on the state of AOS and POL in children with ARP was determined as follows (Tab.5.3).

Table 5.3.

Comparative erythrocyte markers in ARP children before and after treatment.

AOS indicators analysed	Statis strateg ic indicat ion bodies	Control group	ARP before treatme nt	ARP after treatmen t Scheme A	ARP after treatme nt Scheme B
superoxide dismutase units/mg protein	M±m	11.32±0 .16	9.53±0. 42	10.98±0. 21*	9.68±0. 78
glutathione peroxidase mM/min gr protein	M±m	2.02±0. 15	1.84±0. 02	2.13±0.0 9*	1.89±0. 12
catalase µCat/mg protein	M±m	42.08±1 .5	36.48±1 .72	41.32±0. 01*	38.10±1 .8
glutathione reductase mM/min gr protein	M±m	1.68±0. 12	1.35±0. 04	1.56±1.6 *	1.51±0. 08
Nitric oxide µmol/L	M±m	31.02 ±0.12	68.06 ± 8.16	42.02 ± 0.07*	56.15 ± 4.12
glutathione transferase mM/min gr protein	M±m	3,65±0. 02	2.33±0. 11	3,80±0.2 1*	2.07±0. 91*

cytochrome C-oxidase µmol/mg protein	M±m	1.63±0.04	1.33±0.04	1.58±0.09*	1.38±0.11

*p<0.05 - reliability compared to the period before treatment

In children with ARP when treated with melatonin, compared with the period before treatment, AOS parameters increased with treatment regimen A ($P < 0.05$), and nitric oxide decreased to normal levels. Overall, patients who received pathogenetic therapy showed an increase in AOS parameters compared with patients who received conventional treatment. Children who received conventional treatment had a less significant increase in marker concentration.

We have witnessed that melatonin can serve as a broad-spectrum antioxidant (activation of antioxidant pathways). The additional addition of a melatonin-containing preparation to the complex treatment resulted in an increase in the activity of antioxidant enzymes in the blood, such as total superoxide dismutase, glutathione peroxidase, glutathione reductase and catalase. This process is accompanied by a decrease in oxidation in the respiratory chain, eventually leading to a decrease in total malonaldehyde and DA levels. In the study of plasma POL parameters, it was found that DC and MDA levels were elevated in all forms of ARP before treatment. In children with ARP after melatonin treatment, compared to the period before treatment, POL parameters significantly decreased ($P<0.01$; $P<0.05$) (Tab.5.4.).

Table 5.4.

Plasma POL parameters in ARP children before and after treatment.

Analysed groups of children	Analysed parameters of POL (mmol/ml)	
	MDA	DK

Control group	2.68±0.20	1.48±0.11
ARP before treatment	3.68±0.23	1.85±0.08
ARP after treatment Scheme A	2.55±0.05*	1.56±1.2*
ARP after treatment Scheme B	3.25±0.18	1.74±0.27

*p<0.01 - reliability compared to the period before treatment

Thus, the protective effect of melatonin is to increase the activity of antioxidant enzymes including superoxide dismutase, catalase, glutathione peroxidase, glutathione reductase and cytochrome C-oxidase by increasing the expression of the aforementioned enzymes.

Thus, the antioxidant properties of melatonin are based on stimulation of the main antioxidant enzymes, inhibition of NO synthase, reduction of peroxidation products and reduction of free radical formation. It can be said that this mechanism of action of melatonin is related to its neuroprotective effects.

The antioxidant effects of melatonin are related to its biorhythmological and normalising effects on sleep and on endogenous peptide levels.

CONCLUSION

Affective-respiratory paroxysms are a common type of non-epileptic seizure, mainly occurring in infants and young children. They have the ICD-10 code R06, which refers to symptoms without a specific diagnosis.

This causes sudden cerebral ischaemia, inducing an anoxic seizure. Episodes are usually brief and last from 15 s to a minute. ARP usually occurs between 6 months and 3 years of age. The prevalence is estimated to be 1 in 1000 and is more common in boys. Other terms such as white breath-holding and pale infantile syncope are also used to describe ARP, whereas the term "severe breath-holding episodes" is preferred in the North American literature

Currently, the main causes of ARP in children aged six months to four or five years are attributed to the fact that in early childhood many structures of the central nervous system (CNS) are functionally underdeveloped and not fully adapted to the autonomic nervous system (ANS).

This is primarily due to the persistent myelination of nerve fibres after birth. Thus, in children, the spinal cord and its roots are completely covered with myelin sheath only by the age of three, the vagus nerve (vagus nerve) by the age of four, and the axons of the pyramidal pathways of the medulla oblongata by the age of five. But the tone of the vagus nerve stabilises much later, which is probably why affective spasms in newborns are very common.

In early childhood, the sympathetic and parasympathetic section of the ANS, which provides respiration and all other unconditional reflexes, continues to improve. At the same time, the number of nerve impulse transmission synapses increases rapidly, and the excitation of neurons is still sufficiently counteracted by their inhibition, because the child in the subcortex of the brain is insufficient synthesis of gamma-aminobutyric acid (GABA) - an inhibitory neurotransmitter. In early childhood predisposing factors contribute to high nervous excitability and hypertonus sympathetic section of the autonomic nervous system, which is especially active in stressful situations. The excessive reactivity of some structures of the limbic system, in particular, the control of the ANS of the hypothalamus and the hippocampus of the brain, which regulates emotions, also plays its role.

It should be noted that, in contrast to foreign, many domestic paediatricians equate affective spasms in children with hysterical attacks, that is, in fact, a manifestation of hysterical neurosis.

The main risk factors or triggers of ARP in children are: sudden fear, sharp pain, occurring suddenly, for example, when falling, as well as violent expression of negative emotions, stress or nervous-stress shock.

Psychologists have recognised the importance of parents' reactions to their children's strong emotions, irritability or frustration. It is worth remembering that the tendency to such attacks, as well as to many other fainting attacks, can be transmitted genetically - together with the type of autonomic nervous system (hypersympathicotonic or vagotonic).

In addition, possible factors that can provoke breath-holding when a baby cries include iron deficiency anaemia in children.

Thus, early diagnosis of affective-respiratory paroxysms and adequate therapy lead to seizure control, which prevents the development of epileptic seizures, syncopal states and neuropsychiatric disorders in children.

Purpose of the study. Identification of clinical, neurophysiological and pathogenetic features of ARP with the development of proposals and recommendations for optimisation of diagnosis and therapy.

The study is based on the survey data of 103 children with ARP treated in the inpatient department of TashPMI clinic for the period from 2019 to 2021.

The mean age of children with ARP was 13.3 ± 7.2 months (boys 69 (66.9%), girls 34 (33.0%), while in the control group it was 20.9 ± 6.4 months (12 (60%): 8 (40%) (sex ratio 1.5:1), respectively.

The study included analysis of anamnestic and clinical data, neurological examination with the inclusion of neuropsychodiagnostic tests (Pantyukhina G.V., Pechora K.L., Frucht E.L. (2007)), neurophysiological studies (EEG), neuroimaging studies (neurosonography of the brain). The content of biochemical markers (malonic dialdehyde (MDA) and diene conjugates (DC), superoxide dismutase (SOD), glutathione peroxidase, glutathione reductase, catalase, cytochrome C-oxidase and nitric oxide (NO)) in blood serum was determined.

When analysing the data of obstetric and gynaecological anamnesis, pregnancy in women in 85.4% of cases was accompanied by genital and extragenital pathology. The most common pathologies were iron deficiency anaemia during pregnancy (85.4%), toxicosis during pregnancy (56.3%), risk of pregnancy termination (25.2%), pathological course of pregnancy (44.6%), spontaneous abortion in the history (34.9%), infectious and inflammatory diseases of the mother during pregnancy (28.1%), cardiovascular disease of the mother (7.8%) and exacerbation of chronic nasopharyngeal infection (14.5%). Percentage study of obstetric and gynaecological history in the study shows that perfect pregnancy and delivery were very rare.

When analysing the birth status of the studied children using individual medical records, the following clinical cases were identified: 44 (42.7%) babies were born in satisfactory condition, 51 (49.5%) babies were born in moderate condition and 5 (4.9%) babies were born in severe condition. When analysing the gestational age of the children, the following was found: 73 (71%) newborns were premature, 27 (26.2) were premature and 3 (2.9%) were preterm.

The role of indicators assessed by the Apgar scale in the first 5 minutes was analysed in the development of ARP. In this case, in 49 children of the main group the Apgar scale was 7-8 points, in 47 children 5-6 points (mild asphyxia), and in 4 children 3-4 points (medium level of asphyxia), which reflected to what extent the infants' brain hypoxia was in the first minutes.

When studying the neonatal period (the child's condition during the newborn period), 85% of children had perinatal CNS damage of hypoxic genesis (in the form of cerebral excitability syndrome, cerebral depression syndrome, motor dystonia syndrome, vegeto-visceral disorders syndrome and liquor-vascular distention syndrome), 25 per cent had intrauterine dystrophy (hypotrophy), 28 per cent had perinatal (intrauterine) infection and 8 per cent had jaundice before 1 month of age.

As a result of our research, concomitant somatic pathology was registered in 90.2% of ARP children. Pathology of the respiratory system, pathology of the cardiovascular system and gastrointestinal tract were the most frequently observed.

Diseases of respiratory and ENT organs were detected in 48.5% of patients, among which the most frequently registered were out-of-hospital bronchopneumonia (37.6% of patients) and acute rhinosinusitis (11.9% of patients).

Among the diseases of the gastrointestinal tract organs, acute and chronic gastroduodenitis (35.6%), biliary dyskinesia (15.4%) and dysbacteriosis (56.7%) were most frequently detected in patients with ARP.

Analysis of the results of the study showed that of 23.8% of patients with confirmed pathology of the cardiovascular system, sinus node dysfunction was the most frequent - sinus tachy- and bradyarrhythmias in 11.5% of patients, transient atrioventricular (AV) block of the first degree and (AV) block of the second degree were detected equally often in 12.4% of cases in children of the main groups.

The combination of several pathologies was more frequent in the main group of children and accounted for 66.8 %, while in the control group the combined pathology was significantly less frequent and accounted for 5 % ($p < 0.05$).

When studying the family history, we obtained information taking into account the hereditary condition of ARP, where we found that 23% of children in the main group had a paternally aggravated heredity. 77% of hereditary anamnesis was not aggravated.

When examining anamnesis data, the frequency of affective-respiratory paroxysms in 52.4% of children began at the age of 3-12 months, in 29.1% of children at the age of 13-24 months, and in 18.4% of children it was noted that seizures occurred at the age of 25-36 months.

In the research work, we divided the children of the main group into the following forms depending on the nature of the paroxysm. As can be seen from the table, the cyanotic form of ARP was more diagnosed in 45.6% of children, the pale form - in 21.3% of children and the mixed form - in 33.0% of children.

Depending on the severity of the course of ARP attacks, patients were divided into 3 subgroups (mild-33%, moderate-29.1%, severe-19.4%).

When studying the clinical and neurological characteristics of patients with ARP, syndromes characteristic of central nervous system lesions in the perinatal period were identified. The syndrome of increased neuro-reflex excitability in the cyanotic form of ARP was found in 12 (11.6%) children, and in the mixed form of ARP cerebrastenic syndrome was detected with equal frequency.

Clinical and neurological examination of children in the main group revealed the following neurological symptoms: in 3 (2.9%) children strabismus, in 4 (3.9%) children convergence disorders, in 7 (6.8%) children nasolabial folds smoothing, in 3 (2.9%) children slight tongue deviation, in 27 (26.2%) children muscular hypotonia, in 23 (22.3%) children muscular dystonia, 16 (15.5%) children had muscle hypertonia, 36 (34.5%) children had increased deep tendon reflexes, 14 (13.6%) children had suppression of deep tendon reflexes, and 9 (8.7%) children had instability in the Romberg pose.

Psychomotor development disorders were manifested by delayed cortical functions. Delay of cortical functions was marked by the child's lack of interest in toys and others, poverty of emotions, delays in speech and fine motor skills. When testing the function of active speech in (33.9%) children, (understanding of addressed speech) in (15.5%) children of the main group there was a delay of 1 epicrisis term. In the study of sensory development (visual and auditory orienting response) in (11.6%) children of the main group there was a delay of 1 epicrisis term. Children with ARP who scored significantly low on the "emotional sphere" indicator took a long time to come out of any negative emotional state, even when they were comforted by their mothers. This, of course, forced their parents to take drastic measures to please them. The groups of control children could be easily distracted from their bad moods and they responded better to their mother's calls during play compared to the ARP children ($p>0.05$). So, we hypothesise that children with ARP have a 'tendency to stay' in their peak emotional states. Our study clearly showed that respiratory carriers differ from other children in that they are more sensitive, react sharply and intensely to any negative environment. At diagnostics the acquisition of social skills: development of the ability to play (25,2%), constructive activity (11,6%) and pictorial activity (26,2%) of children was formed with a lag of 1 epicrisis term in relation to children of the comparison group ($p>0,05$).

We evaluated the initial vegetative tone in children using A.M. Vein's table. A change in any type of autonomic tone can affect the development of clinical signs of ARP. When assessing the initial vegetative tone, eutonia was registered in 27 children, sympathicotonia in 45 children and vagotonia in 15 children.

At estimation of vegetative reactivity of children of the main group with the help of telt-test it was found out: in 35 (33,9%) children hypersympathicotonic vegetative reactivity, in 15 (14,5%) children asympathicotonic vegetative reactivity and in 50 (48,5%) children normotonic vegetative reactivity, normotonic vegetative reactivity was found out in all children of the control group.

In 58.9% of children with ARP, various brain lesions were detected by NSG. The most frequently detected changes on NSG data were: dilation of the external or internal liquor spaces (36.8%), asymmetry of the lateral ventricles (18.4%), widening of the interhemispheric gap (17.4%), subatrophic changes in the brain substance (15.5%), and lenticulostriary vasculopathy (1.9%).

Children with ARP had significantly lower α-rhythm frequencies in all age groups. The main disturbances of bioelectrical activity in the range of α-rhythm 4.5-7.13 Hz, generalised bursts of slow-wave activity, mainly in the central leads, against the background of normal electrical activity remained. Thus, in our study, asymmetry was recorded in children with ARP in 32%% (n=33). Generalised bilateral-synchronous bursts of high-amplitude θ-, δ-waves, predominantly expressed in the central parietal in 12 (11.6%) children, parieto-occipital in 21 (20.4%) children were detected. According to the frequency of θ- and δ-rhythms, we obtained the following results: in healthy children these indices are 4.73±0.16 and 1.73±0.14, respectively, and in children with ARP - 6.15±0.1 and 2.2±0.12, respectively.

In our study, we evaluated EEG indices depending on the severity of paroxysms. To determine the relationship between the severity of paroxysms and the indices of bioelectrical activity of the brain. Thus, 14.5% of children with mild forms of ARP showed age normal, 13.7% of children showed signs of dysfunction of nonspecific medial brain structures, and the remaining 5.8% of children showed diffuse changes in brain bioelectrical activity in the form of disorganisation of the α-rhythm.

In 34.5% of children with severe ARP, there was a generalised high-amplitude slowing of EEG activity at 4-5 Hz (θ-band), followed by an increase in brainwave amplitude with a decrease in frequency at 1.5-3 Hz (δ-band).

In 14.1% of patients with moderately severe forms of ARP, there was a generalised slowing of high-amplitude EEG in the θ-band, followed by an increase in brainwave amplitude and slowing in the δ-band. This was followed by a sudden decrease in brainwave amplitude, resulting in the disappearance of brain activity ("flat" EEG). Returning to the supine position neither immediately resolved the EEG abnormalities nor restored consciousness, both of which occurred after an additional time interval (mean total syncope duration 41.4 seconds).

Returning to the supine position resulted neither in immediate elimination of EEG abnormalities, but complete normalisation of brain activity occurred after an additional time interval (mean duration 15.1±6.0 seconds; range 7 to 22 seconds). The prevalence of tonic-clonic twitches during loss of consciousness was significantly higher in patients with pale forms of ARP (20 of 22; 90.9%) compared with patients with cyanotic forms of ARP (14 of 46; 30.4%, P<0.01). In all cases, no spike or spike-wave activity, lateralising or focal abnormalities could be detected in any child.

At the end of the test, the EEG was found to be normal in all cases, and no epileptic abnormality was noted in any patient despite the occurrence of syncopal episodes.

The results of the study of lipid peroxidation processes in blood plasma in ARP children showed that MDA and DC levels in mild course show up to the levels of control values (p<0.01), in patients with moderate and severe clinical course these indices are significantly higher (p<0.001) than in control children. Analysing the data, it can be noted that in ARP the concentration of MDA and DC, is a marker of lipid peroxidation. The products of lipid peroxidation lead to damage of the vascular wall, which can cause microcirculation disorder in tissues.

In the metabolism of every cell, an oxidation reaction takes place. The presence of oxygen in the internal environment is, on the one hand, important for cell function; on the other hand, it is a threat that causes oxidative damage due to the formation of free radicals. SOD activity was decreased in the blood of the examined children, while SOD protein levels remained stable compared to the healthy groups. In addition, the decrease in SOD activity was more pronounced in severe ARP than in those with mild ARP.

The study of antioxidant defence parameters revealed their decrease. The content of AOS parameters in blood plasma in children of the main group decreased as the severity of ARP attacks increased ($p<0.01$). These data show that in patients with ARP the content of AOS enzymes in blood was reduced, the amount of POL products was increased, indicating cell membrane damage.

These facts may be due to the fact that oxidative stress products can cause damage to brain cells, which can lead to the development of paroxysms.

During the study, it was noted that the level of cytochrome c-oxidase in serum turned out to be diagnostically significant in predicting affective-respiratory paroxysm. The amount of cytochrome C-oxidase was significantly decreased in severe ARP compared to its mild form ($p<0.01$). Based on this, we can predict that decreased cytochrome C-oxidase levels exacerbate seizures may also lead to epileptic seizure.

We studied the content of nitric oxide metabolites in blood plasma to identify risk factors for the development of ARP. A significant increase in the content of NO metabolites was noted in children of the main group ($p=0.025$), which also indicated the presence of marked cerebral hypoxia. Given its unique characteristics of vasodilation (improvement of blood flow and oxygen supply) and modulation of energy metabolism, nitric oxide (NO) is the main signalling and effector molecule mediating the body's response to hypoxia. We have identified a key role for NO in the adaptation of the organism to an acute mismatch in energy demand.

Micronutrient deficiency to some extent provokes the development of ARP. For this purpose, a general blood analysis of patients was performed to detect iron deficiency anaemia. Total erythrocyte haemoglobin averaged 80.5±4.2 in children of the main group, while in the control group this index was 108.6±3.52, mean erythrocyte count was 3.02±0.1 and 3.85±0.09, mean colour index was 0.78±0.01 and 0.98±0.04. The listed indices are statistically reliable ($p<0.01$).

As a result of blood analysis, iron deficiency anaemia of the II degree was detected in 18 children with severe ARP, in 12 children with moderately severe ARP, and in 5 children with mild ARP. Iron deficiency anaemia of I degree was detected in 68 children.

Our studies have shown that changes in AOS and POL parameters in blood in young children with ARP form the pathophysiological basis for the development of non-epileptic paroxysms, can be an additional diagnostic criterion and have prognostic value for epileptic seizures.

CONCLUSIONS

1. Premorbid factors (obstetric and gynaecological aggravation (85.4%), hereditary predisposition (23%), the consequence of perinatal CNS damage (85%), somatic pathology (90.2%)) in the pathogenesis of affective respiratory paroxysms were revealed. Perinatal hypoxia in combination with aggravated heredity predisposes to an earlier onset of the disease.

2. Clinical and neurophysiological features of ARP were characterised by polymorphism of symptoms and syndromes, depending on the severity of the consequences of perinatal CNS damage. Disturbance of psychomotor development was manifested by delayed sensory (15.5%), speech (33.9%) and fine motor skills (36.8%).

3. Conditions associated with increased oxidative stress in ARF are a risk factor for the development of seizure readiness and may be an additional diagnostic criterion and have prognostic significance. In addition, decreased levels of cytochrome-C-oxidase exacerbate seizures may also lead to epileptic seizure. A significant increase in the content of NO metabolites was noted in children of the main groups (p=0.025), which also indicated the presence of pronounced cerebral hypoxia.

4. The state of lipid peroxidation processes and antioxidant defence system may play a role in the pathophysiology of ARP attacks. Our data indicate that the value of oxidative stress was significantly higher in children with ARP than in controls.

5. Inclusion of melatonin in the treatment complex as an antioxidant drug, promotes inclusion in the system of brain defence

against oxidative stress, selectively prevents free-radical processes, has an antioxidant effect and is an alternative to anticonvulsant therapy in non-epileptic paroxysms.

PRACTICAL RECOMMENDATIONS

1. The task of practical health care is the prevention of perinatal pathology, timely diagnosis, treatment and prevention of possible long-term consequences.

2. Based on the obtained data, it will allow to expand the existing ideas about the role of erythrocyte and plasma markers of the oxidative system in the pathogenesis of ARP, as well as to consider them as prognostic indicators of epilepsy.

3. It was found that combined therapy with melatonin is optimal in children with ARP than traditional therapy of ARP, i.e. it provides improvement of clinical, neurological and metabolic parameters.

Annex 1

Дифференциальная диагностика АРП и эпилепсии

Признаки	**АРП**	**Эпилепсия**
Возраст клинических проявлений	В среднем 6-18 месяцев	Любой возраст
Провоцирующие факторы	Боль, укол, испуг, разочарование, гнев, страх	Отсутствуют
Наследственность	Отягощен	Отягощена
Аура	Отсутствует	Характерна
Приступы во время сна	Отсутствуют	Возможно
Виды приступа	Кратковременные в виде закатывания или замирания	Генерализованный тонико-клонический характер
Время появления цианоза/бледности	на фоне продолжительного крика возникает изменение кожных покровов	Цианоз после потери сознания
Мышечное напряжение	Характерны	После потери сознания
Прикусывание языка и недержание мочи	Не характерно	Характерна
Продолжительность приступа	Менее одной минуты	Более одной минуты
Нарушение ритма сердца	Брадикардия или асистолия при белом типе задержки дыхания	Тахикардия в период приступа эпилепсии
Постиктальная спутанность сознания	Отсутствует	Характерна
Результаты ЭЭГ	Диффузные изменения биоэлектрической активности	Острые высокоамплитудные волны, спайки
Результаты НСГ	Функциональные нарушения	Органические нарушения
Коморбидность	Характерны	Не характерно

Annex 2

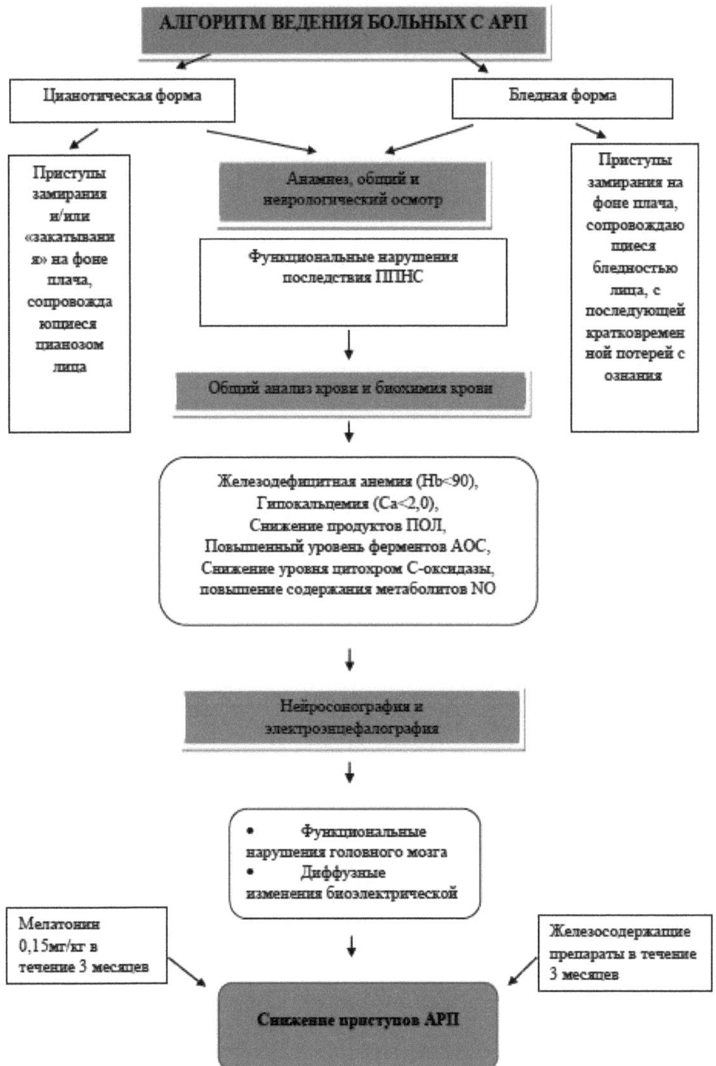
АЛГОРИТМ ВЕДЕНИЯ БОЛЬНЫХ С АРП
Цианотическая форма
Бледная форма
Приступы замирания и/или «закатывания» на фоне плача, сопровождающиеся цианозом лица
Анамнез, общий и неврологический осмотр
Приступы замирания на фоне плача, сопровождающиеся бледностью лица, с последующей кратковременной потерей сознания
Функциональные нарушения последствия ППНС
Общий анализ крови и биохимия крови
Железодефицитная анемия (Hb<90),
Гипокальцемия (Ca<2,0),
Снижение продуктов ПОЛ,
Повышенный уровень ферментов АОС,
Снижение уровня цитохром С-оксидазы,
повышение содержания метаболитов NO
Нейросонография и электроэнцефалография
• Функциональные нарушения головного мозга
• Диффузные изменения биоэлектрической
Мелатонин 0,15мг/кг в течение 3 месяцев
Железосодержащие препараты в течение 3 месяцев
Снижение приступов АРП

REFERENCE LIST

1. Babadjanova U., & Majidova Y. (2022). Delay of psychomotor development in children on the background of somatic aggravation. Journal of Hepato-Gastroenterological Research, 2(3), 64-66.

2. Belousova E.D. Afferent-respiratory seizures//Vrachu-2011, no. 8: 59-61.

3. Voronina T.A. Pantogam and Pantogam active. Clinical application and fundamental research. M. 2009, 11-30.

4. Globa O.V. Neurochemical aspects of convulsive paroxysms in children // Ros. paediatr. zhurn. - 2002. - №5. - C. 31-35.

5. Goryachev S.K., Avdeeva T.I. Clinic and treatment of paroxysmal anxiety-phobic disorders // Journal of neurology and psychiatry. - M., 2007. - №11. - C. 66-67.

6. Guzeva V.I. Epilepsy and non-epileptic paroxysmal states in children. Moscow: Medical Information Agency. 2007. 268 c.

7. Gorbacheva F.E., Chuchin M.Y. Paroxysmal states of non-epileptic nature in childhood. MED-LIBRARY Psychiatry and Psychopharmacotherapy. P.B. Gannushkin №01-Appendix 2004.

8. Dimario FJ, Burleson JA. Autonomic nervous system function during severe breath-holding. Paediatr Neurol. 1993;9: 268-74.

9. Zavadenko N.N. [et al] Cognitive and paroxysmal disorders in the remote period of craniocerebral trauma in children and adolescents: a review / / // S. S. Korsakov Journal of Neurology and Psychiatry: Media Sphere Publishing. - 2019. - Vol. 119 N 1. - C. 110-117 (Cipher Zh3/2019/Volume 119/1).

10. Ziyakhodjaeva L.U., Tozhikhonov N.B. Electroencephalographic changes in cerebrovascular diseases with epileptic paroxysms // Neurology. - Tashkent, 2011. - N4. - C. 123.
11. Kolkiran A., Tutar E., Atalay S., Deda G., Qing S. Autonomic nervous system functions in children with respiratory arrest and iron deficiency outcomes. *Acta Paediatr.* 2005 г.; 94 (9): 1227-1231.
12. Kiseleva L.G., Pyankova M.G. Affective respiratory attacks in children: a modern view of the problem. Paediatria im. G.N. Speransky. 2022; 101 (1): 155-160.
13. Nikanorova M.Yu., Belousova E.D., Ermakov A.Yu. Pseudoepileptic (hysterical) paroxysms in children / M.Y. Nikanorova, E.D. Belousova, A.Yu. Ermakov // Ros. vestnik perinatologii i paediatria. - M., 2001. - №4. - C. 42-46.
14. Palchik A.B. Poniatishin A.E. Non-epileptic paroxysms in infants // ME Dpress Inform. -M.2015. -C. -136
15. Polskaya A. V., Chutko L.S. V., Chutko L.S. Emotional disorders in children with affective-respiratory paroxysms and their mothers // Neurological Bulletin. Journal of V.M. Bekhterev. Kazan: Kazan "Medicine". - 2019. - Vol. LI Issue. 2. - C. 61-65 (Cipher H4/2019/Volume LI/Volume 2).
16. Polskaya A. V. V., Chutko L.S., Yakovenko E.V. Application of the drug pantogam syrup in the therapy of affective-respiratory paroxysms in infants // Journal of Neurology and Psychiatry named after S. S. Korsakov. - M., 2016. - Vol. 116 N8. - C. 74-76.
17. Polskaya A. V., Chutko L.S. V., Chutko L.S. Emotional disorders in children with affective-respiratory paroxysms and their mothers // Neurological Bulletin. - Vol. LI, No. 2 (2019). - C. 61-65.

18. Prokhorova A. V., Tuichieva N.M. V., Tuichieva N.M. Clinical and electroencephalographic picture of paroxysms in children with posttraumatic epilepsy // Neurology. - Tashkent, 2010. - N4. - C. 48-51.

19. Studenikin V. M. Epilepsy in childhood // Lechachashchy Doctor. - M., 2015. - N1. - C. 24-28.

20. Subbarayan A., Ganesan B., Anbumani J. Temperamental traits of children with breath-holding behaviour: a case-control study. *Indian J. Psychiatry.* 2008 г.; 50 (3): 192-196.

21. Eliachik K, Bolat N, Kanik A, et al. Parental attitudes, depression, maternal anxiety, family functioning, and breath-holding: a case-control study. *J. Paediatr. Child Health.* 2016; 52 (5): 561-565.

22. Y.N. Majidova, U.T. Babadjanova Neurological disorders in somatic diseases in young children // Bulletin of KazNMU. 2016. №2.

23. Ali A. Tufail, Jamil M.K., et al. Comparative Analysis of Ethylene/Diene Copolymerisation and Ethylene/Propylene/Diene Terpolymerization Using Ansa-Zirconocene Catalyst with Alkylaluminum/Borate Activator: The Effect of Conjugated and Nonconjugated Dienes on Catalytic Behavior and Polymer Microstructure. Molecules 2021, 26, 2037.

24. Arain AM, Song Y, Bangalore-Vittal N, Ali S, Jabeen S, Azar NJ. Long term video/EEG prevents unnecessary vagus nerve stimulator implantation in patients with psychogenic nonepileptic seizures. Epilepsy Behav. 2011 Aug;21(4):364-6. doi: 10.1016/j.yebeh.2011.06.003.

25. Ashby W.R. An introduction to cybernetics. - London, 1957.
26. Azab SF, Siam AG, Saleh SH, Elshafei MM, Elsaeed WF, Arafa MA, Bendary EA, Farag EM, Basset MA, Ismail SM, Elazouni OM. Novel Findings in Breath-Holding Spells: A Cross-Sectional Study. // Medicine (Baltimore). 2015 Jul;94(28):e1150. doi: 10.1097/MD.0000000000001150.
27. Azman Iste F, Tezer Filik FI, Saygi S. SREDA: A Rare but Confusing Benign EEG Variant. // J Clin Neurophysiol. 2019 Aug 5. doi: 10.1097/WNP.0000000000000623
28. Baumgartner C, Pirker S. Video-EEG. Handb // Clin Neurol. 2019;160:171-183. doi: 10.1016/B978-0-444-64032-1.00011-4.
29. Barriuso B., Astiasarán I., Ansorena D. A review of analytical methods measuring lipid oxidation status in foods: A challenging task. Eur. Food Res. Technol. 2013. P. 1-15.
30. Bettini L, Croquelois A, Maeder-Ingvar M, Rossetti AO. Diagnostic yield of short-term video-EEG monitoring for epilepsy and PNESs: a European assessment. Epilepsy Behav. 2014 Oct;39:55-8. doi: 10.1016/j.yebeh.2014.08.009.
31. Buyukgoz C, Mendez MD. Breath Holding Spells. StatPearls [Internet]. Treasure Island (FL): StatPearls Publishing; 2020-.2019 Nov 11.
32. Calik M, Ciftci A, Sarikaya S, Kocaturk O, Abuhandan M, Taskin A, Kandemir H, Yoldas TK, Aksoy N. Assessment of both serum S-100B protein and neuropeptide-levels in childhood breath-holding spells. Epilepsy Behav. 2015 Jun;47:34-8. doi: 10.1016/j.yebeh.2015.04.039.

33. Carman KB, Ekici A, Yimenicioglu S, Arslantas D, Yakut A. Breath holding spells: point prevalence and associated factors among Turkish children. //Pediatr Int. 2013 Jun;55(3):328-31. doi: 10.1111/ped.12090.

34. Chaves-Carballo E. Syncope and paroxysmal disorders other than epilepsy. InPedi-atric Neurology: Principles & Practice. Eds: Swaiman KF, Ashwal S, Ferriero DM.4th edition. Philadelphia, PA, Mosby-Elsevier, 2006.

35. Chen L, Knight EM, Tuxhorn I, Shahid A, Lüders HO. Paroxysmal non-epileptic events in infants and toddlers: A phenomenologic analysis. Psychiatry Clin Neurosci. 2015 Jun;69(6):351-9. doi: 10.1111/pcn.12245

36. Cokar O, Gelisse P, Livet MO, Bureau M, Habib M, Genton P. Startle response: epileptic or non-epileptic? The case for "flash" SMA reflex seizures. Epileptic Disord. 2001 Jan-Mar;3(1):7-12.

37. Cross J. Pitfalls in the diagnosis and differential diagnosis of epilepsy // Pediatrics and child health.-2009.-Vol.19.-P.199-203.

38. Dai AI, Demiryürek AT. Effectiveness of Oral Theophylline, Piracetam, and Iron Treatments in Children With Simple Breath-Holding Spells. J Child Neurol. 2020 Jan;35(1):25-30. doi: 10.1177/0883073819871854.

39. Daoud A.,Batieha A., Al-Sheyyab M. et al. Effectiveness of iron therapy on breath-holding spells //Journal of Pediatrics. - 1997.-Vol.130.-P.547-550.

40. De Myer W. Breath-holding spells. Current management in child neurology.- 3nd ed. -London, 2005. - P353-355.

41. Desai SD, Desai D, Jani T. Role of Short Term Video Encephalography with Induction by Verbal Suggestion in Diagnosis of Suspected Paroxysmal Nonepileptic Seizure-Like Symptoms. Epilepsy Res Treat. 2016;2016:2801369.

42. Di Mario F.J., Burleson J.A. Autonomic nervous system function in severe breath-holding spells // Pediatric Neurology.-1993.-Vol.9.N4; 268-274.

43. Di Mario F. Prospective study of children with cyanotic and pallid breath-holding spells //Pediatrics. -2001.-Vol.107.- P.265-269.

44. Donma M. Clinical efficacy of piracetam in treatment of breath-holding spells //Pediatric neurology. - 1998. - Vol.18. - P. 41-45.

45. Ergul Y, Otar G, Nisli K, Dindar A. Permanent cardiac pacing in a 2.5 month-old infant with severe cyanotic breath-holding spells and prolonged asystole. Cardiol J. 2011;18(6):704-706. PubMed PMID: 22113764.

46. Fernández-Alvarez E. Transient benign paroxysmal movement disorders in

infancy. // Eur J Paediatr Neurol. 2018 Mar;22(2):230-237.

47. Ferretti A, Barresi S, Trivisano M, Ciolfi A, Dentici ML, Radio FC, Vigevano F, Tartaglia M, Specchio N. POGZ-related epilepsy: Case report and review of the literature.//J Med Genet A. 2019 Aug;179(8):1631-1636. doi: 10.1002/ajmg.a.61206.

48. Feyissa AM, Tatum WO. Adult EEG.andb Clin Neurol. 2019;160:103-124. doi:10.1016/B978-0-444-64032-1.00007-2.

49. FRANCIS J. DIMARIO, JR., MD. Non-Epileptic Childhood Paroxysmal Disorders. Oxford University Press, Inc., publishes

works that further Oxford University's objective of excellence in research, scholarship, and education. 2009; 39-40.

50. Ghossein J, Pohl D. Benign spasms of infancy: a mimicker of infantile epileptic disorders. Epileptic Disord. 2019 Dec 1;21(6):585-589. doi: 10.1684/epd.2019.1116.

51. Gonzalez Corcia MC, Bottosso A, Loeckx I, Mascart F, Dembour G, François G. Efficacy of treatment with belladonna in children with severe pallid breath-holding spells Cardiol Young. 2018 Jul;28(7):922-927. doi: 10.1017/S1047951118000458.

52. Goraya J.S. Treatment of cyanotic breath-holding spells with oral theophylline in a 10-year-old boy. //J of Child Neurol.2015;30:919-921.

53. Huang LL, Wang YY, Liu LY, Tang HP, Zhang MN, Ma SF, Zou LP. Home Videos as a Cost-Effective Tool for the Diagnosis of Paroxysmal Events in Infants:Prospective Study. JMIR Mhealth Uhealth. 2019 Sep 12;7(9):e11229. doi:10.2196/11229.

54. Holmes GL, Sackellares JC, McKiernan J, et al. Evaluation of childhood pseudoseizures using EEG telemetry and videotape monitoring. J Pediatr 1980;97;554-558.

55. Irmen F, Wehner T, Lemieux L. Do reflex seizures and spontaneous seizures form a continuum? - triggering factors and possible common mechanisms. //Seizure. 2015 Feb;25:72-9. doi: 10.1016/j.seizure.2014.12.006

56. Ito Y, Kidokoro H, Negoro T, Tanaka M, Okai Y, Sakaguchi Y, Ogawa C, Takeuchi T, Ohno A, Yamamoto H, Nakata T, Maesawa S, Watanabe K, Takahashi Y, Natsume J. Paroxysmal

nonepileptic events in children with epilepsy. Epilepsy Res. 2017 May;132:59-63. doi: 10.1016/j.eplepsyres.2017.02.009.
57. Kartal A. Paroxysmal Tonic Upgaze in Children: Three Case Reports and a Review of the Literature. Pediatr Emerg Care. 2019 Apr;35(4):e67-e69. doi: 10.1097/PEC.0000000000001327.
58. Kholi H, Vercueil L. Emergency room diagnoses of psychogenic nonepileptic seizures with psychogenic status and functional (psychogenic) symptoms: Whopping. // Epilepsy Behav. 2020 Mar;104(Pt A):106882. doi: 10.1016/j.yebeh.2019.106882.
59. Klepper J, Leiendecker B, Eltze C, Heussinger N. Paroxysmal Nonepileptic Events in Glut1 Deficiency. // Mov Disord Clin Pract. 2016 Nov-Dec;3(6):607-610.doi: 10.1002/mdc3.12387.
60. Koontz EH, Hanson J, Pritchard PB 3rd. Diagnostic outcomes of inpatient video electroencephalography: nonepileptic events in South Carolina. J S C Med Assoc.2013 Sep;109(3):82-4.
61. Kubik A, Mitkowska Z, Kwinta P, Skowronek-Bała B, Kaciński M. [The role of videoelectroencephalography in diagnostics of seizures in neonates and infants].// Przegl Lek. 2005;62(11):1236-43.
62. Lawley A, Manfredonia F, Cavanna AE. ideo-ambulatory EEG in a secondary care centre: A retrospective evaluation of utility in the diagnosis of epileptic and nonepileptic seizures. // Epilepsy Behav. 2016 Apr;57(Pt A):137-140. doi: 10.1016/j.yebeh.2016.02.005..
63. Lněnicková D, Makovská Z, Lněnicka J. [Affective respiratory and reflex

Paroxysms-evaluation of anamnestic data, clinical manifestations and therapy].Cesk Pediatr. 1993 Aug;48(8):477-480. Czech.

64. Metrick ME, Ritter FJ, Gates JR, et al. Nonepileptic events in childhood. Epilepsia 1991; 32; 322-328.

65. Montenegro MA, Eck K, Jacob S, Cappell J, Chriboga C, Emerson R, Patterson MC, Akman CI. Long-term outcome of symptomatic infantile spasms established by video-electroencephalography (EEG) monitoring. J Child Neurol. 2008 Nov;23(11):1288-92. doi: 10.1177/0883073808318540

66. Morgan LA, Dvorchik I, Williams KL, Jarrar RG, Buchhalter JR. Parental ranking of terms describing nonepileptic events. Pediatr Neurol. 2013 May;48(5):378-82. doi: 10.1016/j.pediatrneurol.2012.12.029.

67. Müller MJ, Paul T. [Syncope in children and adolescents] //Herzschrittmacherther Elektrophysiol. 2018 Jun;29(2):204-207. doi:10.1007/s00399-018-0562-2.

68. Nagy E, Hollody K. Paroxysmal non-epileptic events in infancy: five cases with typical features.//Epileptic Disord. 2019 Oct 1;21(5):458-462. doi: 10.1684/epd.2019.1098.

69. Naud J. [Apparent life-threatening events and sudden unexpected death in infancy: Two different entities]// Arch Pediatr. 2015 Sep;22(9):1000-4. doi: 10.1016/j.arcped.2015.05.021.

70. Nechay A, Stephenson JB. Bath-induced paroxysmal disorders in infancy. Eur J Paediatr Neurol. 2009 May;13(3):203-8. doi: 10.1016/j.ejpn.2008.04.004.

71. Orivoli S, Facini C, Pisani F. Paroxysmal nonepileptic motor phenomena in newborn. Brain Dev. 2015 Oct;37(9):833-9. doi: 10.1016/j.braindev.2015.01.002.

72. Ozbay OE. Idiopathic paroxysmal tonic upward gaze. Pediatr Neurol. 2012 Oct;47(4):306-8. doi: 10.1016/j.pediatrneurol.2012.05.028.

73. P. T. Popławski and R. A. Derlacz, [How does melatonin function?] [Article in Polish] Post. Biochem. 49 (2003) 1-9.

74. Paech C, Wagner F, Mensch S, Antonin Gebauer R. Cardiac pacing in cardioinhibitory syncope in children. Congenit Heart Dis. 2018 Nov;13(6):1064-1068. doi: 10.1111/chd.12682.

75. Qubty W, Renaud DL. Cognitive impairment associated with low ferritin responsive to iron supplementation. Pediatr Neurol. 2014 Dec;51(6):831-3. doi: 10.1016/j.pediatrneurol.2014.08.035.

76. Rathore G., Larsen P., Fernandez C., Parakh M. Diverse presentation of breath-holding spells: two case reports with literature review //Case Repotrs in Neurological Medicine.-2013.-Article ID 603190.-P.1-3.

77. Ristić AJ, Mijović K, Bukumirić Z, Vojvodić N, Janković S, Baščarević V, Đukić T, Sokić D. Differential diagnosis of a paroxysmal neurological event: Do neurologists know how to clinically recognise it? Epilepsy Behav. 2017 Feb;67:77-83. doi: 10.1016/j.yebeh.2016.12.022.

78. Repetto, Marisa, et al. 'Lipid Peroxidation: Chemical Mechanism, Biological Implications and Analytical Determination'. Lipid Peroxidation, InTech, Aug. 2012. Crossref, doi:10.5772/45943.

79. Reiter R. J. et al. Melatonin defeats neurally-derived free radicals //J. Physiol. Pharmacol. - 2007. - VOL. 6. - P. 5-22.
80. Reiter R. J. et al. Obesity and metabolic syndrome: association with chronodisruption, sleep deprivation, and melatonin suppression //Annals of medicine. - 2012. - T. 44. - №. 6. - C. 564-577.
81. Reiter R. J. et al. Reducing oxidative/nitrosative stress: a newly-discovered genre for melatonin //Critical reviews in biochemistry and molecular biology. - 2009. - T. 44. - №. 4. - C. 175-200. 227
82. Reiter R. J. Pineal melatonin: cell biology of its synthesis and of its physiological interactions //Endocrine reviews. - 1991. - T. 12. - №. 2. - C. 151-180.
83. Reiter RJ, Acuña-Castroviejo D, Tan DX, Burkhardt S. Free radical-mediated molecular damage. Mechanisms for the protective actions of melatonin in the central nervous system. Ann N Y Acad Sci. 2001 Jun;939:200-15. PMID: 11462772.
84. Robinson JA, Bos JM, Etheridge SP, Ackerman MJ. Breath Holding Spells in Children with Long QT Syndrome.// Congenit Heart Dis. 2015 Jul-Aug;10(4):354-61. doi: 10.1111/chd.12262.
85. Roddy S.M. Breath-holding spells and reflex anoxic seizures. In:Swaiman K.F., Ashwal S., Ferriero D.M.et al, eds.// Swaiman's Pediatric Neurolofy:Principles and Practice.6th ed. Philadelphia,PA:Elsevier,2017.chap85.
86. Roubertie A, Leydet J, Soete S, Rivier F, Cheminal R, Echenne B. [Non epileptic paroxysmal movement disorders in childhood]. Arch Pediatr. 2007 Feb;14(2):187-9

87. Sakaue S., Chiyonobu T., Morotoel M., et al. A case with recurrent asystole dut to breath-holding spells:successful treatment with levetiracetam //No To Hattatsu. - 2012. - Vol.44.- P.496-498.

88. Sanabria-Castro A, Henríquez-Varela F, Monge-Bonilla C, Lara-Maier S, Sittenfeld-Appel M. Paroxysmal events during prolonged video-video electroencephalography monitoring in refractory epilepsy. Neurologia. 2019 May;34(4):234-240. doi: 10.1016/j.nrl.2016.12.003

89. Sawchuk T, Buchhalter J. Psychogenic nonepileptic seizures in children - Psychological presentation, treatment, and short-term outcomes. Epilepsy Behav. 2015 Nov;52(Pt A):49-56. doi: 10.1016/j.yebeh.2015.08.032.

90. Sirman Y.V., Savitsky I.V., Price N.I. Dynamics of malonic dialdehyde level in experimental diabetic retinopathy and methods of its correction. Actual problems of modern medicine. Volume 20, Issue 4 (72). C. 95-100.

91. Stechyshyn, I., Pavliuk, B. et al. (2020). The quercetine containing drugs in pharmacological correction of experimental diabetes with myocardial injury. Romanian Journal of Diabetes Nutrition and Metabolic Diseases, 26(4), 393-399.

92. Tyazhka O.V., Zagorodnya Ya. M. The state of lipid peroxidation and antioxidant system in children of different ages. Perinatology and pediatrics. no. 2. 2016. pp. 101-105. https://doi.org/10.15574/PP.2016.66.101

93. Shih JJ, Fountain NB, Herman ST, Bagic A, Lado F, Arnold S, Zupanc ML, Riker E, Labiner DM. Indications and methodology for

video-electroencephalographic studies in the epilepsy monitoring unit.// Epilepsia. 2018 Jan;59(1):27-36. doi: 10.1111/epi.13938.

94. Shuper A., Mimouni M. Problems of differentiation between epilepsy and non-epileptic paroxysmal events in the first year of life //Arch.Dis. Child. - 1995.-Vol 73. - P.342-344.

95. Silbert P.L., Gubbay S. Familial cyanotic breath-holding spells // J. Pediatr. Child. Health. 1992. Vol. 28 (3):254-256.

96. Sohal AP, Khan A, Hussain N. Prolonged video-EEG in identifying paroxysmal nonepileptic events in children with epilepsy: a useful tool. J Clin Neurophysiol. 2014 Apr;31(2): 149-51. doi: 10.1097/WNP.0000000000000035.

97. Stewart LS. Endogeneous melatonin and epileptogenesis: Facts and hypothesis. The International Journal of Neuroscience. 2001;107:77-85

98. Steward LS, Leung LS. Hippocampal melatonin receptors modulate the seizure threshold. Epilepsia. 2005;46:473-480

99. Sousa L, Gonorazky S. [Paroxysmal upgaze deviation syndrome]. Arch Argent Pediatr. 2010 Oct;108(5):e108-10. doi: 10.1590/S0325-00752010000500012

100. Szabó L, Siegler Z, Zubek L, Liptai Z, Körhegyi I, Bánsági B, Fogarasi A. Adetailed semiologic analysis of childhood psychogenic nonepileptic seizures. // Epilepsia. 2012 Mar;53(3):565-70. doi: 10.1111/j.1528-1167.2012.03404.x.

101. Tarodo SG, Nguyen T, Ranza E, Vulliémoz S, Korff CM. A triad of infantile spasms, nystagmus and a focal tonic seizure. // Epileptic Disord. 2018 Aug 1;20(4):295-300. doi: 10.1684/epd.2018.0984.

102. Thomas AA, Preston J, Scott RC, Bujarski KA. Diagnosis of probable psychogenic nonepileptic seizures in the outpatient clinic: does gender matter? // Epilepsy Behav. 2013 Nov;29(2):295-7. doi: 10.1016/j.yebeh.2013.08.006.
103. Verducci C, Friedman D, Devinsky O. SUDEP in patients with epilepsy and nonepileptic seizures. // Epilepsia Open. 2019 Jun 6;4(3):482-486. doi: 10.1002/epi4.12342. eCollection 2019 Sep
104. Verrotti A, Trotta D, Blasetti A, Lobefalo L, Gallenga P, Chiarell F. Paroxysmal tonic upgaze of childhood: effect of age-of-onset on prognosis. Acta Paediatr. 2001 Nov;90(11):1343-5
105. Vigevano F, Fusco L, Pachatz C. Neurophysiology of spasms. Brain Dev. 2001 Nov;23(7):467-72. Review.
106. Visser A., Jaddoe V., Arends L., et al. Paroxysmal disorders in infancy and risk factors in population-based cohort: the Generation R.Study//Dev.Med.Child.Neurol.-2010.-Vol.52. - P.1014-1020.
107. Vurucu S, Karaoglu A, Paksu SM, Oz O, Yaman H, Gulgun M, et al. Breath holding spells may be associated with maturational delay in myelination of brain stem.// J Clin Neurophysiol. 2014;31:99-101.
108. Venkataraman P. et al. Effect of melatonin on PCB (Aroclor 1254) induced neuronal damage and changes in Cu/Zn superoxide dismutase and glutathione peroxidase-4 mRNA expression in cerebral cortex, cerebellum and hippocampus of adult rats //Neuroscience research. - 2010. - T. 66. - №. 2. - C. 189-197.
109. Vigneri P. et al. Diabetes and cancer //Endocrine-related cancer. - 2009. - T. 16. - №. 4. - C. 1103-1123.
110. Vinogradova I., Anisimov V. Melatonin prevents the development of the metabolic syndrome in male rats exposed to

different light/dark regimens //Biogerontology. - 2013. - T. 14. - №. 4. - C. 401-409.

111. Vivekananthan D. P. et al. Use of antioxidant vitamins for the prevention of cardiovascular disease: meta-analysis of randomised trials //The Lancet. - 2003. - T. 361. - №. 9374. - C. 2017-2023. 232

112. Wade A. G. et al. Nightly treatment of primary insomnia with prolonged release melatonin for 6 months: a randomised placebo controlled trial on age and endogenous melatonin as predictors of efficacy and safety //BMC medicine. - 2010. - T. 8. - №. 1. - C. 51.

113. Wade A. G. et al. Prolonged release melatonin in the treatment of primary insomnia: evaluation of the age cut-off for short- and long-term response //Current medical research and opinion. - 2011. - T. 27. - №. 1. - C. 87- 98.

114. Waldhauser F. et al. Alterations in nocturnal serum melatonin levels in humans with growth and aging //The Journal of Clinical Endocrinology & Metabolism. - 1988. - T. 66. - №. 3. - C. 648-652.

115. Wang X. M. et al. Effects of perindopril on soluble intercellular adhesion molecule-1 in patients with congestive heart failure //Heart. - 2002. - T. 88. - №. 4. - C. 417-417.

116. Wang X. S. et al. Shift work and chronic disease: the epidemiological evidence //Occupational medicine. - 2011. - T. 61. - №. 2. - C. 78-89.

117. Ware Jr J. E. SF-36 health survey update //Spine. - 2000. - T. 25. - №. 24. - C. 3130-3139.

118. Wade A. G. et al. Nightly treatment of primary insomnia with prolonged release melatonin for 6 months: a randomised placebo

controlled trial on age and endogenous melatonin as predictors of efficacy and safety //BMC medicine. - 2010. - T. 8. - №. 1. - C. 51.

119. Walsh M., Knilans T., Anderson J., Czosek R. Successful treatment of pallid breath-holding spells with fluoxetine //Pediatrica.-2012.-Vol.130.-P.e685-e689.

120. Wang B, Cai FC. [Clinical and polyneuroelectrophysiological characteristics of infantile spasm]. Zhonghua Er Ke Za Zhi. 2007 Feb;45(2):109-14.

121. Wei D, Garlinghouse M, Li W, Swingle N, Samson KK, Taraschenko O. Utilization of brain imaging in evaluating patients with psychogenic nonepileptic spells.//Epilepsy Behav. 2018 Aug;85:177-182. doi: 10.1016/j.yebeh.2018.06.015.

122. Wichaidit BT, Østergaard JR, Rask CU. Diagnostic practice of psychogenic nonepileptic seizures (PNES) in the paediatric setting. //Epilepsia. 2015 Jan;56(1):58-65. doi: 10.1111/epi.12881.

123. Ya.N.Madjidova, U.T. Babajanova, V.K.Abdullaeva, Sh.A.Shirmatov, Khalilova A.A. Affective-respiratory paroxysms in children: clinical-neurological aspects. European Journal of Molecular & Clinical Medicine 7 (2), 2020.

124. Yadav D, Chandra J. Iron deficiency: beyond anemia // Indian J Pediatr. 2011 Jan;78(1):65-72. doi: 10.1007/s12098-010-0129-7.

125. Yilmaz U, Doksoz O, Celik T, Akinci G, Mese T, Sevim Yilmaz T. The value of neurologic and cardiologic assessment in breath holding spells // Pak J Med Sci. 2014 Jan;30(1):59-64. doi: 10.12669/pjms.301.4204.

126. Yilmaz O, Ciftel M, Ozturk K, Kilic O, Kahveci H, Laloğlu F, Ceylan O. Assessment of heart rate variability in breath holding

children by 24 hour Holter monitoring. // Cardiol Young. 2015 Feb;25(2):317-23. doi: 10.1017/S1047951113002333

127. Yoshinaga H, Kobayashi K, Endo F, Ishizaki Y, Wakai M, Ohtsuka Y. Abnormal fast activity in infancy with paroxysmal downwards gaze. Brain Dev. 2009 Jun;31(6):435-41. doi: 10.1016/j.braindev.2008.08.007.

128. Zehetner A., Orr N., Buckmaster A., et al. Iron supplementation for breath-holding attacks in children // Cochrane Database Syst Rev. - 2010; 12, (5) CD008132.

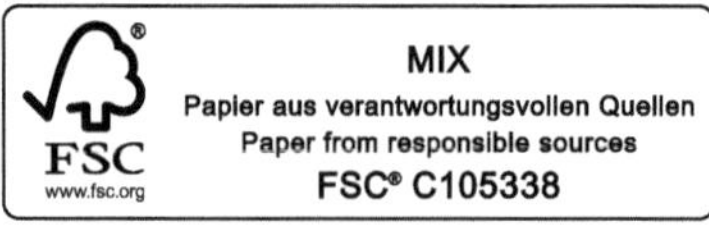

Printed by Books on Demand GmbH, Norderstedt / Germany